HOW TO BE A
ROCK
STAR
DOCTOR

THE COMPLETE GUIDE TO
TAKING BACK CONTROL OF YOUR LIFE
AND YOUR PROFESSION

REBEKAH BERNARD, MD

Book Layout and Cover Design: www.PearCreative.ca

Print: 978-0-9964509-0-4
eBook: 978-0-9964509-1-1

To the many wonderful patients who have allowed me to share in their lives, and for my mom, who always wanted to be a "fly on the wall."

THE ROCK STAR RULES

1. Anytime you are with a patient, remember that you are "on-stage"

2. When in doubt, ask yourself: "Is this in the best interest of my patient?"

3. Be available

4. Listen to your patients

5. Learn how to show empathy

6. Make the 'Problem List' your best friend

7. Learn to document an exam just by looking

8. Health maintenance: Every visit, every time

9. Maximize patient-physician face-to-face time

10. You don't need to know all the answers, just where to *find* them

11. Don't sell yourself short!

12. Make your mental health a priority

CONTENTS

CHAPTER ONE   11
Why you'll love becoming a Rock Star doctor:

CHAPTER TWO   15
Getting on-stage or: Playing the role of "Doctor"

CHAPTER THREE   19
Background and street cred

CHAPTER FOUR   23
What is a Rock Star physician?

CHAPTER FIVE   27
Finding your audience

CHAPTER SIX   29
Rock Star availability

CHAPTER SEVEN   35
Create availability by Rock Star scheduling

CHAPTER EIGHT   39
Managing challenges in the schedule

CHAPTER NINE   47
Use the schedule to prevent physician burn-out

CHAPTER TEN   49
The "affable" doctor

CHAPTER ELEVEN   53
Qualities of the Rock Star physician

CHAPTER TWELVE   67
The Rock Star scene: Setting the stage

CHAPTER THIRTEEN   81
The Rock Star team

CHAPTER FOURTEEN   91
The Rock Star debut – Getting "on-stage"

CHAPTER FIFTEEN   99
Listening or 'Six seconds to Rock Star"

CHAPTER SIXTEEN   107
Empathy and demonstrating interest

CHAPTER SEVENTEEN   111
Establish and develop the patient's agenda

CHAPTER EIGHTEEN   115
Using a Problem List to develop the physician agenda

CHAPTER NINETEEN   123
Rock Star secrets:

CHAPTER TWENTY   127
The gynecologic exam or "Get in, get out"

CHAPTER TWENTY-ONE   131
Explaining the diagnosis and communicating the treatment plan

CHAPTER TWENTY-TWO   137
The initial patient visit

CHAPTER TWENTY-THREE   141
Health Maintenance

CHAPTER TWENTY-FOUR   143
The wellness visit and screening codes

CHAPTER TWENTY-FIVE   153
Getting off-stage

CHAPTER TWENTY-SIX   157
The importance of follow-up visits

CHAPTER TWENTY-SEVEN   161
Office flow and maximizing patient-physician face-to-face time

CHAPTER TWENTY-EIGHT   167
Controlled substance prescribing

CHAPTER TWENTY-NINE   171
Dealing with lab results – "No news is not good news!"

CHAPTER THIRTY   175
Prior authorizations and other forms

CHAPTER THIRTY-ONE   181
Clinical challenges in medicine – Rock Star solutions

CHAPTER THIRTY-TWO   189
Clinical issues - Dealing with challenging patients

CHAPTER THIRTY-THREE   201
Managing the challenging patient

CHAPTER THIRTY-FOUR   209
The truly hateful patient

CHAPTER THIRTY-FIVE   213
Patient dismissals

CHAPTER THIRTY-SIX   219
Death and dying – the terminally ill patient

CHAPTER THIRTY-SEVEN   223
Finding the answers

CHAPTER THIRTY-EIGHT   225
Using evidence-based medicine (EBM)

CHAPTER THIRTY-NINE   227
The peripheral brain

CHAPTER FORTY   235
Finding the answers:

CHAPTER FORTY-ONE   237
Practice, practice, practice

CHAPTER FORTY-TWO   241
Working with consultants and the medical team

CHAPTER FORTY-THREE   249
Managing hospitalizations

CHAPTER FORTY-FOUR   257
Rock Star charting

CHAPTER FORTY-FIVE 261
Rock Star charting secrets – efficient note-writing techniques

CHAPTER FORTY-SIX 269
Computer tips and tricks – surviving the electronic record

CHAPTER FORTY-SEVEN 273
Office procedures and wound care

CHAPTER FORTY-EIGHT 281
Billing and coding tips for Rock Star office visits

CHAPTER FORTY-NINE 291
Mental health for physicians

CHAPTER FIFTY 299
Special stresses for women physicians

CHAPTER FIFTY-ONE 305
Finding work-life balance and satisfaction

CHAPTER FIFTY-TWO 311
Rock Star physician practice options

CHAPTER FIFTY-THREE 319
Advocacy

CHAPTER FIFTY-FOUR 323
Conclusion

ACKNOWLEDGEMENTS 329

BIOGRAPHY OF CONTRIBUTORS 331

ENDNOTES 333

FORMS 349

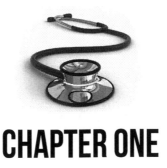

CHAPTER ONE

WHY YOU'LL LOVE BECOMING A ROCK STAR DOCTOR:

YOU CAN TAKE BACK CONTROL OF YOUR LIFE AND YOUR PROFESSION

Are you facing some or all of these cringe worthy physician pain points?

- Accountable Care Organization (ACO)
- Meaningful Use (MU1, 2, 3…)
- Electronic Health Record (EMR)
- Maintenance of Certification (MOC)
- "Value Based Care" (PQRS, etc)
- Alternative Payment Model (APM)
- Merit-based Incentive Payment System (MIPS)

If you shuddered as you were reading this list with its alphabet soup of abbreviations, you may be one of the 46% of practicing physicians who reported feeling burned out from the profession of medicine. If not, give it time – after all, only 40% of docs reported feeling burned out two years ago, with the number experiencing burnout only expected to increase.[1]

Physician burnout is a serious problem. The practice of medicine has become increasingly stressful; in addition to actual medical care, which has become ever more complex with advancing science and technology, physicians have been forced to navigate an unprecedented political and economic climate.

Just take a look at a sampling of programs above that physicians have been forced into over the last few years. Each requires an enormous amount of work and expense on the part of the physician, despite the lack of clear scientific evidence that any of them benefit the health care system.

And this increased stress has taken its toll on physicians. Burnout leads to a constellation of negative consequences, causing harm not only to physicians in the form of increased depression, alcohol abuse, and suicide, but also to our patients through decreased quality of care, increased medical errors, and a decreased physician work-force.[2]

Whether you're just starting your journey in residency or you're a seasoned pro, you may be experiencing burnout, struggling to remember why you wanted to become a physician in the first place. Charting and never-ending paperwork may be just starting to beat you down, or perhaps you've resigned yourself to a life of prior authorizations, declining reimbursement, and 10-minute visits while fantasizing about the unlikely possibility of an early retirement.

Good news: There is a way to take back control of your life and your profession. The secret lies in learning to become a Rock Star Physician!

The results: Get out of work earlier, spend less time on needless documentation, and make your patients happier by following the rules of Rock Star physicians. Using these simple strategies, you will learn to modify your "on-stage" behavior to get the most out of each patient encounter, maximizing profit while improving patient satisfaction, and protecting yourself from burnout and compassion fatigue.

Learn the secrets and "work-arounds" that the busiest and most in-demand physicians use to create an organized, efficient, and positive patient experience:

- Convey the qualities that are the most important to patients, leading to clinical success
- Organize and control the office visit to maximize the patient and physician agendas
- Optimize time management by the use of clinical tools such as the "Problem List" and Evidence-Based-Medicine (EBM)
- Focus on physician-patient "face-to-face" time to maximize profitability
- Overcome the challenges of the Electronic Health Record (EHR) on the physician-patient relationship with time-saving methods such as customizable forms
- Cope with emotionally challenging patients by learning to show empathy, even when you don't feel it
- Use psychology to maintain your mental health and find work-life balance

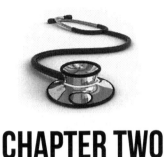

CHAPTER TWO

GETTING ON-STAGE OR: PLAYING THE ROLE OF "DOCTOR"

Remember the first time you put on your white lab coat and ID badge, draping that brand-new Littmann stethoscope around your neck? Like me, you may have felt like an imposter "playing" doctor, a sensation that would follow you from one clinical rotation to the next. For some of us, that sense of being an imposter has never really left.

Which makes sense. Think about it: After seven or eight years of rigorous training, we developed the knowledge and skills to diagnose and treat disease; but at what point did we learn how to truly play the part of doctor? Little formal training on how to practice is provided in medical school curricula. And much of our residency programs are essentially "on-the-job training" as we emulate senior residents or just stumble along through trial and error.

Relationships are everything in medicine, and yet most of our medical school patient experience is limited to brief bedside encounters in the hospital setting, usually at 5 AM while the patient is half asleep! While creating a strong physician-patient relationship is the cornerstone to clinical success, we are provided with little of the tools and practice that we need to hone this critical skill during our training years.

And what about learning to practice medicine in "the real world," outside of the sheltered hospital walls of tertiary care and academia? While most of us will go on to practice medicine outside of urban medical centers, we rarely have an opportunity to experience an environment not dominated by academic medicine during our training.

In our first jobs outside of training, we face a sharp learning curve – not only are we practicing medicine on our own for the first time, but we have to figure out logistics that we never considered before: What resources are available in our new community; who are the best (or only!) subspecialists; how do we get our patients admitted to the local hospital? That's not to mention suddenly facing the business and financial aspects of medical care and running a practice.

Medical training focuses on the science of medicine, but experience and real life teaches you the art and business of medicine.

"It is different to practice medicine than it is to learn to be a doctor," says Paul Marsolek, an expert on Physician Performance Improvement. "Years of study are different from applied learning." And years of study in academic medicine can be significantly different from real world medicine.

While there is no substitute for volume and experience, this book shares with you years of wisdom from highly successful practicing clinical physicians, breaking down an ideal practice into ten simple rules, starting with the most basic:

During my training, the most useful advice on playing the "role" of doctor came from Douglas Meuser, MD, my attending physician and first Rock Star physician mentor: "Always remember that you are on-stage."

At that time in my career, the concept of on-stage meant trying not to "let 'em see you sweat" – much more "Fish Bowl" than Rock Star. I would try to "act" like a doctor in front of patients, like nodding and saying "mm-hmm," in my best TV doctor inflection during the physical exam. Or I would BS my way through patient questions when I didn't know the answer and then step out of the exam room to look things up or to get advice from a more senior physician.

It took years for me to gain an understanding of the importance of being on-stage, but it has now become my guiding mantra and the true secret of becoming a Rock Star doctor.

Being on-stage is much more than "acting" like a doctor by just trying to project an appearance of confidence and composure in front of patients. It means demonstrating a demeanor of care and concern, when those might be the last emotions that you are feeling inside. It involves "directing" the patient experience in a way that makes a ten-minute visit seem to the patient that you spent much longer.

Being on-stage means standing up for your convictions when it would be so much easier to give in. It means making your patients believe you and believe in you. And it means knowing how to get "off-stage" to prevent burnout and compassion fatigue.

While on-stage, the Rock Star physician uses techniques that maximize productivity while maintaining the highest standard of medical care. These techniques also lead to high patient satisfaction, lower liability risk, and overall improvement in physician job satisfaction.

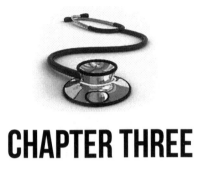

CHAPTER THREE

BACKGROUND AND STREET CRED

So what gives me the "street cred" to write an advice book for physicians, and in particular, the chutzpa to call myself a Rock Star? The simple answer: my patients think that I am.

How do I know? Volume and patient feedback.

For the last 10+ years, I have consistently been the most "productive" primary care physician in the two multi-physician groups with whom I have worked. But, I have also had the highest patient satisfaction scores. This combination earned me the top 1% of RVUs and salary based on MGMA standings for primary care physicians.

And when I recently decided to open my own solo practice, the vast majority of my patients followed me and I was so inundated with requests for new patients that I had to close my panel within just a few months of the move.

And where did I come up with this Rock Star concept?

At my last position as a hospital-employed physician, I received quarterly patient satisfaction scores and feedback. A few years ago I received a patient review that read: "Dr B. is a Rock Star!" My first response was to shake my head and laugh at such a crazy idea, but then I started to ponder…what would make a physician a "Rock Star?"

Paul Marsolek, former director of Loyalty, Engagement, and Performance Improvement at Health Management Associates, put it this way: "You are the busiest primary care physician in the practice, yet you received the highest satisfaction scores, in particular for the patient response 'My doctor spent time with me.' How is that possible?"

How to deliver top performance and top patient satisfaction results: By following the Rock Star Rules.

Over the last 15 years, I've played the role of physician in multiple settings and I have learned that the Rock Star Rules are universal. They worked for me during my seven years serving the very poorest patient populations with multiple cultural and language barriers – as well as with the "affluenza"-stricken suburban set -- 5 years in an area of the highest concentration of millionaires (interestingly within the same county).

The rules work in rural Federally Qualified Health Centers caring for patients with minimal to no literacy, as well as in for-profit hospital systems working with some of the most educated members of society – retired physicians, PhDs, and former Fortune 500 CEOs.

And the Rules can work in any setting that *you* choose - most recently I have created my own niche as a solo physician practicing primary care in an Urgent Care setting, where I see the spectrum of non-obstetrical

Family Medicine - caring for newborn babies up to the most senior citizens. Guess what? The Rules still apply.

The Rock Star Rules also help physicians to navigate one of the most challenging aspects of medicine – medical records. Having worked extensively with multiple Electronic Health Records (Epic, Centricity, NextGen, AllScripts, Suncoast, and LytecMD) as well as several years on paper, I have learned tips, tricks, and work-arounds to make charting a less painful experience. In fact, every company I have worked for has relied on me as a "go-to" for my less tech-savvy physician colleagues.

And yes, I've made mistakes. I've experienced both what to do and also what *not* to do. So I will share some of those mistakes. Part of becoming a Rock Star doctor is acknowledging our own humanity, while critically analyzing medical errors and using them for better patient care in the future. Like many physicians, I have struggled with my own psychological wellness, which I have learned to prioritize to achieve both personal and professional success.

I've also spent a great deal of time among colleagues who are Rock Stars in their own right, collecting their common characteristics and shared behavior patterns. I have interviewed some of the busiest, most in-demand physicians – mentors, colleagues, and leaders both in the "Ivory Tower" and in the "trenches" to gather the tips and secrets that make them loved by their patients.

And in addition to expert opinion and recommendation, I have scoured the scientific literature to provide evidence-based solutions for the most common challenges in providing medical care today.

We all went into medicine with the goal of "helping people." Somewhere along the line, the time crunches and minutiae of the "health care system" may have distracted us. We, as physicians, can take back control by getting on-stage – learning to practice medicine in a way that will lead to improved patient care and personal job satisfaction.

So that you can develop your own Rock Star physician persona, I will show you how to change from mild-mannered physician to Rock god – at least while you are in the office. You don't have to change who you are – clearly you have outstanding clinical skills and a decent personality to have reached your current level. Instead, learn how to display the attributes that will make your patients love you, while maximizing your income and limiting unproductive office time.

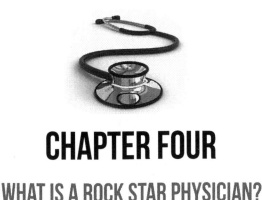

CHAPTER FOUR

WHAT IS A ROCK STAR PHYSICIAN?

Obviously sex, drugs, and rock-n-roll are out of the equation (well, maybe a little rock-n-roll in a really modern office), but many elements of star quality correlate with a physician office.

While I'm dating myself with this reference, my mental images of rock stars follow the "Hair Band" '80s: a charismatic, confident, "front-man" (or woman), for whom the public is willing to shell out big bucks to see in concert, even putting up with hours of a horrible opening band while waiting for the appearance.

Or, to translate Rock Star into the physician analogy: Be a personable doctor whom patients are happy to pay to see and even willing to tolerate a waiting room delay for the privilege. And we don't even have to wear leather pants.

The Rock Star doctor gives his patients what they are looking for and what they expect. She has a great personality that makes her patients feel comfortable and confident. According to Alan Falkoff, MD, a Rock Star physician "has the talent to be empathetic with a wide variety of patients by outward words, appearances, and body language that conveys to the patient that you care for them."

The Rock Star physician is available and ready to perform when patients need him. And, of course, he's damn good at what he does. As Ariel Cole, MD, Family Physician and Medical Director of Florida Hospital's Geriatric Fellowship program says: "A Rock Star doctor balances efficiency with great patient care."

Emily Nabors, MD, Family Physician and winner of 2010's Most Influential Woman and 2011 Patient's Choice Award adds: "A Rock Star physician is not only educationally sound and compassionate, but also has finesse."

So, let's go crazy with this Rock Band analogy. Imagine that we've got our kick-ass rock band together on stage – we've got our lead singer AKA "Rock Star," guitarist, bass player, drummer – the band manager and accountant are off to the side; the stage manager is ready to fire up the pyrotechnics. Everyone is in place; the lights come up and... nothing. No audience. No cheering, screaming fans. No ticket sales.

You get the picture. Without an audience, or in our case, a patient panel, the show cannot go on. A Rock Star physician has to attract *and retain* a great patient following, effectively and efficiently managing a patient panel.

The bottom line in becoming a successful physician, and especially a Rock Star physician, is *never to lose patient focus.* You will never go wrong if you ask yourself: "Is this decision in the best interest of my patient(s)?" Hey, remember, I said this was about being a Rock Star, not a rocket scientist!

ROCK STAR RULE #2:

When in doubt, ask yourself: "Is this in the best interest of my patient(s)?"

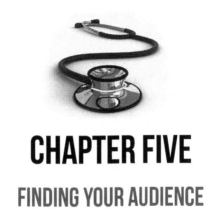

CHAPTER FIVE

FINDING YOUR AUDIENCE

How does a Rock Star doctor develop a great patient following? Medical literature often cites the 3 A's that patients desire in a physician:

Availability

Affability

Ability

It is interesting to note that *ability* is the *least* important characteristic to patients. Whether you graduated Alpha Omega Alpha or barely passed Gross Anatomy (*ahem...*); graduated from Harvard or from a med school deep in the Caribbean, patients don't much care. Remember the old joke: "What do you call the medical student who graduated last in his class? Doctor."

In general, people don't select their physician by considering their clinical acumen. The average patient has to trust that we all know a decent amount of medicine, or at least enough to pass our board certifications, because they really don't have any other option. A patient being able to judge a physician's clinical skills would be like me trying to decide if my mechanic is leading me down the right path or just trying to sell more parts. I have no idea; I just know that my car is making that funny little sound!

So, how does a patient select a physician and how do they decide that this is a "good" doctor? Most of the time, patients tend focus on the first A – *availability*. Or in the case of my car mechanic, I need my car fixed and I need it now!

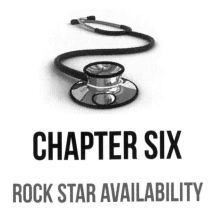

CHAPTER SIX

ROCK STAR AVAILABILITY

ROCK STAR RULE #3:

Be available for your patients

A Rock Star physician must be available for his or her patients. I'm not talking about a 24/7, "here's my cell phone number," type of accessibility, unless a concierge-type service is your goal. But, if your patient calls at 9 AM with a cough and runny nose and you are in the office that day, you need to be able to offer a same-day appointment.

It's a win-win situation: the patient is happily seen by her own doctor and you billed for a quickie upper respiratory infection (URI) visit in between all of your exhaustingly complex chronic medical management. And if insurance reimbursement remains unchanged, you'll probably get paid about the same for the 5-minute URI as your super-sick complicated patients!

The Rock Star physician will see every patient with an acute problem on the same or next day. How? I will show you later that by following the Rock Star rules and cutting back on non-direct patient care hours, you will be freed up to spend your time on what's really important – patient care.

An acute visit can mean *anything that is concerning to the patient.* When in doubt, bring 'em in. An anxious patient is an angry or unhappy patient. Bringing the patient in for a quick check will reassure them and will avoid uncompensated telephone time later on. Emphasize to your staff that sick patients are *never* to be turned away without your knowledge. "I remind my staff that we are here for our patients – they are never a 'nuisance,'" says Dr. Emily Nabors.

The bottom line: physician availability = appointment slots. The reality is that with the traditional payment model, physicians are only compensated for the time we spend in the office or at the bedside of our patient. The only way that we get paid is with an office visit. So, if your patients want to talk with you, they are invited to come into the office for an appointment.

Patient questions, concerns, and clarifications require an office visit.

Family questions and concerns require an appointment. Family members are encouraged to come with patients for their appointments and patients are welcomed to schedule a family meeting as long as the patient is present (required for Medicare billing).

Not only is this policy financially sensible, but it optimizes patient care by providing more face-to-face physician access. An office visit is almost always the best way of evaluating your patient and providing the best medical care. Most patients appreciate the thoroughness of a doctor office visit, and those few who simply want their care on their own terms (via the telephone or email) can seek another physician.

Whether you are employed by a group or are independent, billable encounters are the lifeblood of you and your company's profit margin. No patient encounters = no salary, no staff raises, no electricity.

ROCK STAR TIP:
See your own patients whenever possible

Offering acute office visits is much more than just financial viability. Being available for our patients is our *job*, and is in the best interest of our patients. Our patients *should* have their questions and concerns addressed. They should be examined if they have clinical concerns. And they shouldn't have to resort to using a retail walk-in clinic or emergency department unless there is no other option. As primary care physicians, we are in a better position to treat our own acutely ill patients than a random "doc-in-the-box" retail health center, where patient records are minimal, care is almost always provided by a nurse practitioner (95% in one study[3]), and often information is not communicated back to the primary care physician.

We are also doing ourselves as physicians a disservice when we don't see our own patients, as we may lose patients to competing urgent care centers. The study cited above showed that people who visited such clinics were less likely to return to a primary care physician for future illnesses and also have less continuity of care. Bad for the patient, bad for us.

For the days that you are out of the office, offer patients an appointment for your next clinic day, unless the issue is truly urgent. For those cases, arrange coverage with a trusted colleague or team up with a single good quality urgent care center that sends you records and facilitates follow-up.

In my latest practice setting, I have partnered with an urgent care center staffed by physicians and physician assistants that I trust. On my clinic days, I see all comers. When I am not in the office, my patients have access to one of my colleagues seven days per week, medical records are available to the urgent care staff, and I receive every single office note when my patients are seen so that I can review the treatment plan and arrange follow-up myself.

For this program to work, it is essential to have a strong relationship with your covering physician or urgent care. It is helpful to have one of your staff members available to answer phone calls and facilitate referrals for care when you are not in the office. In my office, we have printed up special identification cards for my patients to present at the urgent care to ensure the best continuity of care.

ROCK STAR TIP:

Don't give away your time

But where do we find the time to see these extra patients? The first step is to eliminate any wasted time in our day and the most important way to do this is to stop giving away physician time on uncompensated labor.

Unlike attorneys, our billing clock only starts ticking when we have a face-to-face encounter with a patient. Phone calls to family members, e-mails, conversations with nursing home directors – at present, none of these services are compensated; even though they may take a considerable amount of physician time that could be better spent with patients in the office.

The only way to be fairly compensated for work as a physician is to see your patients in the office. Therefore, medication refills require an appointment. Lab results require an appointment. Prior authorizations, insurance paperwork, disability forms, disabled parking passes, jury duty medical excuses, school medical excuse notes, and work physical forms require appointments. You get the idea.

Every time a form appears on your desk, forward it to your secretary with a note to bring the patient in for an office visit. The amount of time saved is enormous – while each form may only take a few minutes to fill out, we are so inundated with paperwork that the average physician spends 16% of her time on administrative tasks not related to patients currently in the office.[4] That averages to almost nine hours per week!

I find that doing paperwork while the patient is in the office generally saves time overall – the chart is ready for you, rather than you having to pull it yourself, the patient can directly answer many of the questions that need to be addressed on the form, and the doctor has the opportunity to address care needs that relate to the paperwork, such as changing a medication or requesting prior authorization for a medication that is medically necessary but not covered on the patient's insurance. The doctor gets paid for his time and can therefore pay his electric bill. Win-win.

So now that all of the time that is usually spent on paperwork is freed up, the Rock Star physician has *plenty* of open slots in their schedule for same-day appointments. Your staff should be trained to anticipate and schedule appointments immediately when patients call with questions – you are happy to address all of their needs at their face-to-face visit. "How is today for you?"

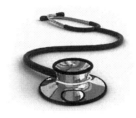

CHAPTER SEVEN

CREATE AVAILABILITY BY ROCK STAR SCHEDULING

There are several philosophies on ideal office scheduling. Traditionally, time is blocked in slots allotted by appointment types: new patients and physicals might get a 40-minute slot, established routine follow-ups 30 minutes, acute work-in visits 15 minutes. A busier practice might "double-" or even "triple-book" any given number of slots, expecting to see a patient every 5-10 minutes such as during cold and flu season or back-to-school physicals.

As discussed above, it is essential to ensure that your schedule allows adequate appointment slots for urgent, acute care visits. These can be dispersed throughout the day or reserved during certain intervals, such as the last hour of the morning or the end of the day.

Emily Nabors, MD, leaves 5-6 available slots in her schedule for work-in, same day appointments. "What's the point in having a physician if you can't see her when you're sick?"

Roberta Chung, MD, former Chief Resident and Rock Star physician agrees. "If you set aside slots for work-ins you can always accommodate someone who wants to be seen that day without throwing your entire schedule off."

The advantage to traditional scheduling is that staff can anticipate and plan for patient needs. And patients, especially retirees, may like to plan their appointments ahead of time. On the other hand, no-shows or cancellations as well as a rush of urgent acute office visits can throw the schedule into complete disarray.

Another paradigm is called "open access" scheduling, in which patients call and are seen on the same day, regardless of the reason for the visit. This type of schedule gives busy working patients more flexibility but may challenge the staff to anticipate patient needs – such as ensuring that paperwork is prepared, insurances verified, etc.

A Rock Star doctor's "routine" schedule can never be set in stone. Like a living thing, the schedule will expand and contract, wax and wane as it is affected by factors such as the school year, summer vacation, and flu shot season. Analyze your schedule critically for scheduling gaps or times that always seem to get overbooked. Don't be afraid to play around with changes. If they don't work, you can always go back to the previous way. A Rock Star doc will always engage staff in schedule decision-making – your office and nursing staff have a totally different perspective and they may see details that are not apparent to you.

If possible, offer a few early morning or later afternoon appointments, or even weekend hours. This is another area that can benefit from creativity and trial and error, depending on your patient population. Working patients and parents are often especially appreciative of consistent, flexible scheduling.

Regardless of the scheduling model, the Rock Star physician will always remember their primary focus: patient care. If you are struggling to accommodate patient demand, first assess how you are spending your office hours. If the physician is performing any non-essential and time-consuming tasks, delegate them to a team member.

Assess any significant drains on the practice such as a staff member not working effectively, a particularly demanding insurance contract with unreasonable administrative burdens or even a handful of extra-difficult patients. These can be enough to affect your office flow and keep you from providing the care that the majority of your patients need. It may make more sense to eliminate those factors than to add extra clinical hours or to stop accepting new patients.

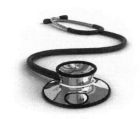

CHAPTER EIGHT

MANAGING CHALLENGES IN THE SCHEDULE

THE "FREQUENT FLYER"

Every doctor has a panel of "frequent flyers" with a multitude of underlying psychological conditions, especially anxiety disorders. These patients tend to show up without appointments, often in crisis, and can severely impact the day's schedule.

The key to managing these patients is to *schedule* frequent follow-up visits. This will cut back on same-day, "urgent" appointments. If your patient knows that he has an appointment with you next week, he may not call in today for reassurance about a non-critical issue.

When I will be out of the office for a few weeks, I try to get my most anxious patients in before I leave, just to touch base, and schedule another appointment for when I return. This minimizes unplanned visits with my covering physician or local emergency room while I am away.

For patients who constantly interrupt your schedule and cause a drain on your staff despite your best efforts, consider ending the relationship. Highly burdensome patients can absorb an immense amount of time, restricting access for others, and creating physician and staff burnout.

NO-SHOWS

A Rock Star physician has minimal no-shows – after all, your patients *want* to see you! However, memories can fail and reminder phone calls or e-mails the day before the appointment make for good office policy.

A missed appointment every now and then is understandable, but habitual no-show-ers should be shown the door with a standardized dismissal letter noting that failure to follow up with visits terminates the physician-patient relationship and jeopardizes patient care. The same goes for habitual late arrivers after they have been gently (and again perhaps not so gently) reminded – unless you come up with an alternate solution that won't trash your schedule.

OVERBOOKING

A Rock Star doctor is worth waiting for, but not forever. Eventually the crowd becomes restless and starts throwing things, which is never good.

The major hazard of being available for your patients is the potential for overbooking. You have to be there when your patient needs you, but how will you know how many patients may need you on any particular day?

While you can make some predictions based on trends, no one can plan for a sudden cold snap that brings out the asthma patients or an uptick in anxiety patients brought on by current political events.

First of all, it is essential that you keep patients informed of wait times. "If you're running late," says Dr. Emily Nabors, "Make sure that your patients know." Your receptionist should advise patients when they check in if the doctor is running on time. If the schedule is really backed up, as in the case of an office emergency, offer the patient the option of rescheduling.

ROCK STAR TIP:

When we reschedule patients, we try to offer them our "best" slot – the first morning appointment or the first afternoon appointment, when it is very rare to be running late. Being late *again* for a rescheduled appointment will really annoy even your most dedicated patients.

When running way behind, it's even better when the doctor himself pokes his head out into the waiting room to apologize for the delay. Patients are far more tolerant of waiting when they don't feel that they have been forgotten. Most patients understand about wait times, especially since they know that whenever it is their turn, no matter how behind the Rock Star physician is, the patient will receive full attention. They also know that if *they* are sick, their physician will be available.

Full disclosure: I often run late in my practice, not uncommonly up to an hour. I hate it – it makes me anxious and I feel badly for making people wait, but it tends to be inevitable no matter how carefully I try to manipulate the schedule. While I am aware that there will always be some type of emergency that crops up during the day, whether I have to call for an ambulance transfer or spend extra time with a patient to give tragic news – it is impossible to predict *when* during the day that will happen, or how many times, making planning for all contingencies an impossibility.

I am in the habit of routinely apologizing for my tardiness (even when I'm on time!), and I never try to "make up" time by rushing patients later in the schedule. My patients know that if I'm behind, it's because I had to spend extra time with someone else – but if *they* ever need extra time, they will get it. Or, like the always late-to-start Rock Star – the concert won't stop until the crowd has heard *all* the hits!

While running behind may be inevitable in a busy practice, there are steps to minimize waiting times. The first is to start your day on time – and preferably a bit early.

ROCK STAR TIP:

Always start 15 minutes early

Sounds like common sense, but this can be a tricky point. For example, your first patient is scheduled at 8 AM and shows up on time, but by the time he does front-desk paperwork, has vital signs measured and data entered into your EHR by your assistant, it may already be 8:20 by the time he is ready for you. Meanwhile, your 8:15 is being readied, and your 8:30 showed up early… you get the drift.

So, instead of starting "on time," imagine the scenario starting fifteen minutes early.

You and your patient show up at 7:45 AM, saying hello in the elevator. The patient was scheduled at 7:45 and is impressed that you see patients so early, as she doesn't have to miss much work. You walk into your office to get the computer up and running, make your coffee, check your in-box… all while your assistant is prepping the patient. At 8 AM the patient is ready and you start your day *on time*. Meanwhile, your next patient is not scheduled until 8:15, so you have a nice little buffer. Do the same thing with your first appointment after lunch.

One of the biggest strains on office flow is lack of critical information needed for the office visit, such as records and results. Any type of computer issue can completely destroy your schedule. So the Rock Star physician must have a contingency plan in place. Start by having your schedule and important patient information ready before you start your workday.

After experiencing several computer crashes, I learned the value of having pre-printed patient information. Most importantly, we always print out our schedule the night before, including patient contact information. There's nothing more frustrating than not being able to at least call your patients to reschedule or advise them of a potential delay in their appointment time.

Your staff should review the patients' charts a day or two before the appointment and ensure that the relevant information is available, such as lab and radiology reports, specialist notes or forms to be filled out. Any relevant information should be printed ahead of time, so it can be reviewed and given to the patient at the visit. Ideally, your clinical assistant should be able to prepare this information for you. "I am lucky to have a Registered Nurse in my office," says Dr. Emily Nabors. "I would never be able to see the volume of patients that I do without her assistance in preparing all of the necessary paperwork."

Ariel Cole, MD, a Geriatric Fellowship Director has the opposite experience. "I end up doing a lot of preparation myself. I would be so much more effective if I had a nurse who could print out the information that I need."

Using a pre-printed schedule also helps your staff to maintain your expectations. Jennifer Keehbauch, MD, 2007 Florida Family Physician of the Year and current president of the Florida Academy of Family Physicians uses the printed schedule to remind her Medical Assistant of tasks that need to be done. "I write notes by each patient's name of things that I would like my assistant to do, such as 'needs repeat urinalysis,' needs flu shot,' etc. This is especially important if the MA is new and doesn't know my rhythm."

ROCK STAR TIP:

Use the patient's last note as a hand-out
CAUTION: Make sure that your office notes are 'patient-friendly!'

It is extremely helpful to print out each patient's last office visit note. Not only is this critical if you lose connectivity to your electronic health record, but you can also use this information to remind yourself, at a glance, of the issues addressed at the last visit, rather than having to open the computer and click through multiple screens.

An additional benefit to printing the last office visit note is that it can also be used to mark any changes in medications or instructions for the follow-up plan. This paper can then be given as a hand-out to the patient at check-out. Since studies show that 40-80% of medical information given by doctors is forgotten immediately[5], the last office note is a great reference when the patient asks herself after leaving the office, "Now what was it that I was supposed to do?"

Also patients can learn more about their health by reading their office notes. I have had many patients return to the next visit and ask things like: "This paper says I have diabetes. Is that true?" even though you are confident that you talked to them about diabetes multiple times.

Remember that more than a third of American adults lack sufficient health literacy to understand their health care[6] and handouts are a great way to help patients to understand the medical plan.

Many patients also appreciate having copies of the notes for their personal medical record or to provide to other physicians.

ROCK STAR TIP:
Capture billing for the "add-on" visit

Add-on unscheduled patients can often cause the physician to run behind, but are an inevitable part of a primary care practice. You know the one – you're in the exam room seeing a well child, when mom points to a sibling and says, "Can you just check little Jimmy's throat? He's been complaining that it hurts."

What are you going to say? No? You'll have to schedule another appointment for Jimmy? Of course not. What kind of heartless monster are you? "I told the doctor that Jimmy was sick and she wouldn't even check him while she was right there!"

So what you *will* do is take a peek at Jimmy's throat, do a quick exam of other relevant body parts while you elicit the history, and make a treatment recommendation, as well as writing a note in the chart.

And you *will* bill for this patient encounter. On your way out, you discreetly murmur to your receptionist (or scribble a note), "Please make a billing ticket for Jimmy," and appropriately code for the level of service provided.

The same goes for husband and wife visits. How many times have you been talking with one member of the couple when the other asks, "Oh, by the way, did you get *my* test results back too?"

"Well let's just take a look," you say cheerfully, even if you are groaning inside. Why? Because most patients don't *get* how this interrupts your schedule and will be disappointed that you didn't answer their request. "I just asked for one little thing while she was right on her computer and she made me schedule an appointment," they will later complain to their friends.

So you might as well suck it up and get paid for your work.

So, when Mrs. Smith commandeers her husband's appointment time for herself, you immediately pull up the patient's chart, review the labs – in detail if time permits, briefly if not, and get a billing ticket from your receptionist. By now, she knows what it means when you say, "I need a ticket for *Mrs.* Smith, too."

If the "add-on" patient's lab results are going to require further investigation, your patient will usually happily accept your advice to schedule a visit "so that we can give this matter the attention it deserves." Most people understand that a detailed explanation requires a visit – they just don't realize that even a brief lab review is going to set the doctor back.

In my experience, most patients don't complain about getting a bill for the add-on experience. If they do inquire about why they got a bill "when you were just seeing my wife," I explain that "You had questions about your health care, and once I open your chart in the computer, it automatically generates an office visit." This is usually accepted– and if the patient is not satisfied with this explanation, he will likely avoid playing add-on in the future or he may choose to find another physician. That's OK too.

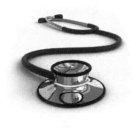

CHAPTER NINE

USE THE SCHEDULE TO PREVENT PHYSICIAN BURN-OUT

While patient care is the Rock Star doc's primary focus, we know that we have to minimize burn-out. To me, one of the very worst things that can affect the morale of a doctor is down-time in the office.

In my first few months transitioning to a new job, my schedule was very light as the word got out and new patients began to trickle in. Sometimes I would only have 2-3 patients per day, often with some thoughtless scheduler putting in one appointment at 8 AM, one at 1 PM, and another at 4:30 PM, and nothing in between! My employer at the time required that I "put in" a full 40 hour week. *Torture.*

I tried *everything* to keep myself busy – organizing my desk, reviewing medical journals, visiting local pharmacies and specialists to market myself, but ultimately there were just too many hours in the day to fill. Once I had proven myself by rapidly rising productivity, I earned some schedule flexibility, but I will never forget those painful weeks and months.

An empowered Rock Star physician will analyze his schedule to maximize productivity and minimize downtime. If Mondays tend to be busy and it slows down by Thursday, do a 10 hour on Monday and knock off early later in the week. If it's important to you to get home early on Fridays, or to come in late on Tuesdays, then make it happen!

Emily Nabors, MD, uses creative scheduling. "I work 9-5 on Monday and Tuesdays, 9-12 on Wednesdays, and 7:30-3pm on Thursday and Friday." This allows her to have time off during the week and also provides early morning appointments for working patients.

In the hot Florida summer when our Northern visitors return home, my schedule slows down significantly. I started experimenting with working three 12-hour shifts per week to keep those days full, maximizing productivity while allowing an additional day free from the office. Interestingly, I found that I could accommodate my routine patient appointments even as work demand grew busier within those three 12-hour shifts – the days are long and intense, but the massive improvement in my quality of life having four days off more than compensated and my staff felt the same way.

Full disclosure: Not all of my patients love my new schedule. While working people, students, and parents love the 7 AM or 6 PM appointment availability, some patients feel anxious that I am not in the office every day and have transferred their care to another physician. That's OK. With the demand for primary care outstripping supply, there are always more patients to be seen. Because I'm happier and less burned-out, I'm a better doctor to the patients who have chosen to stay and with my increased job satisfaction, I no longer fantasize about early retirement, so my patients can keep me longer, too.

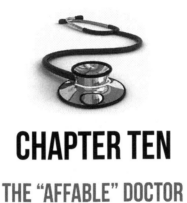

CHAPTER TEN

THE "AFFABLE" DOCTOR

Availability

Affability

Ability

OK, so we've made ourselves available to our patients. Now what? After availability, our patients value "affability" in their physician. Check out the definition of affable from the Merriam-Webster dictionary:

1. Being pleasant

2. Being at ease in talking to others

3. Characterized by ease and friendliness

SYNONYMS

easygoing, breezy, devil-may-care, happy-go-lucky, laid-back, low-pressure, mellow

ANTONYMS

high-strung, uptight

RELATED WORDS

carefree, casual, dégagé, lackadaisical, nonchalant, unaffected, unconcerned, unfussy, unperturbed, untroubled, unworried; familiar, homey (also homy), informal; flexible, lax, lenient, permissive, pliable, pliant, soft; accessible, approachable; imperturbable, nerveless, unflappable, unshakable; amicable, companionable, comradely, cordial, genial, hail-fellow-well-met, hearty, neighborly, warm, warmhearted

NEAR ANTONYMS

ceremonious, decorous, formal, rigid, strict; anxious, bothered, distressed, worried; jittery, jumpy, nervous, skittish, tense

Look at the synonyms and related words – accessible, well, we already hit that one. Easy-going, approachable, warm-hearted, companionable... sounds like someone you'd like to hang out with, doesn't it?

Now look at the antonyms, or opposites: yikes. "High-strung, uptight." Remind you of anyone you went to med school with?

How about "ceremonious, rigid, and bothered." Sounds like the way most TV and movie doctors are depicted!

The Rock Star physician may not be feeling particularly affable on a given day, but can learn to portray these qualities during patient visits.

For example, consider the concept of appearing "untroubled and unworried." We're doctors; we're pretty much *always* troubled. That's kind of our job; to be worried about our patients' problems, isn't it?

Yet our patients want us to walk in as if the only thing on our mind is right there in that exam room and that patient is your one and only concern. He wants to feel that you're not even worried about him, because he's going to be *just fine*. The Rock Star doc makes it feel that way, even if isn't true.

How about the terms "unaffected, unflappable." An affable doctor is supposed to appear nonjudgmental and frankly downright unimpressed with whatever our patients throw at us, even traditionally taboo subjects.

An affable doctor is also seen as "lax, lenient, and flexible." So patients *don't* want us to yell at them when they don't take their meds? Sounds reasonable. Or maybe I should say affable.

The Rock Star doctor doesn't have to actually *be* affable. It helps, but it isn't mandatory. The doc just has to play the part, but play it well. Remember, you are on-stage, and this ain't dinner theater. We have to make our patients believe in us. And that starts by understanding what patients really want from a physician.

So what are the qualities that *patients* think make a Rock Star physician affable?

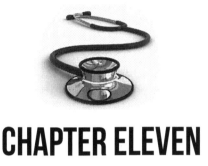

CHAPTER ELEVEN

QUALITIES OF THE ROCK STAR PHYSICIAN

A study in the Mayo Clinic Proceedings asked patients to describe their best and worst experiences with their doctors. The study uncovered seven traits identified as contributing to the ideal doctor: *Empathy, confidence, humanity, personal touch, honesty and forthrightness, respect, and thoroughness.*[7] So, if these are the qualities that patients want, this is what the Rock Star physician is going to give them!

ROCK STAR RULE #4:

Learn to show empathy

The Merriam-Webster dictionary defines empathy as: "the feeling that you understand and share another person's experiences and emotions; the ability to share someone else's feelings."

Empathy is the key to physician-patient communication and is directly related to patient satisfaction, adherence to medical treatment, lawsuits, and clinical outcomes.[8] Empathy is communicating to the patient: "I hear what you are saying, I understand what you are feeling, and I care."

Empathy is the ability to give the *impression* that you understand and care. It's an essential component of the physician-patient relationship. Paul Marsolek, an expert on physician communication, explains it like this: "Empathy is not just a feeling; it's an action, or a verb. Empathy means making a person feel like they are the most important part of the physician's day."

So why do so many physicians struggle with showing empathy?

Studies have shown that students begin medical school with high levels of empathy.[9] This makes sense – most of us start out wanting to alleviate suffering, heal illness, and contribute to society. Unfortunately, empathy is quickly beaten out of us. Medical school, particularly third year clinical rotations, has a catastrophic effect on our levels of empathy.[10]

Theories for this decrease in empathy abound, including the psychological need for medical students to emotionally detach themselves from the amount of pain and suffering witnessed in the hospital setting, to the stress and barriers caused by time pressures, and even to neurotransmitter changes that seem to be required when switching between emotional and analytical thinking.[11]

But while the reason for this significant drop in empathy is not fully understood, studies show that burnout, emotional exhaustion, depression, and cynicism have negative effects on empathy.[12] And the mental strain of training only worsens during our residency years. Studies on internship show that enthusiasm at the beginning of training soon transitions to depression, anger, and fatigue.[13] Eventually, physicians face ongoing erosion of compassion throughout a "career-long battle as pressure to become increasingly efficient squeezes out time for building relationships with patients."[14]

In order to become a Rock Star physician that patients love and trust, we must learn to re-develop some of that empathy that we started out with in medical school. We have to learn to manage the stress associated with disease and suffering in a healthy way, as loss of empathy in med school may actually be a subconscious "maladaptive" response to our own anxieties.[15] When we are anxious, we naturally will have trouble empathizing with our patients. In other words, we probably all need our own personal psychologist (see 'Mental Health' section).

HOW TO DEVELOP EMPATHY: PRACTICE, PRACTICE, PRACTICE

Not everyone is naturally extremely empathetic, even starting out as a first year med student. Fortunately, demonstrating empathy can be learned. As Paul Marsolek, an expert on physician-patient relationships says: "If it's not natural, it has to be learned. Everyone has some empathy – it just isn't always recognizable."

SMILE

One of the easiest ways to demonstrate empathy is by smiling. I always take a deep breath before I enter an exam room and walk in the door with a big smile. I smile as if I am genuinely happy to see the patient (and usually I am, but not always!). I even do this when I am making rounds on my in-patient hospice patients – even when a person is having one of their worst days, a smile can make things a little brighter. "How are you so happy all the time?" my patients ask me. Well, guess what? I'm *not* happy all the time. I might not even be happy right now. But I can act like I am and that goes a long way.

EYE CONTACT

Second easiest way to show empathy: look your patient in the eyes. Now that wasn't so hard, was it?

PERSONAL TOUCH

Different from a "diagnostic touch," such as a physical examination, the personal or social touch increases a patient's perception of physician empathy. A social touch is a handshake, pat on the back or brief hug. [16]

LISTENING

Active listening, using facial expressions, and body language are critical to demonstrating empathy (see later section).

FOSTER CURIOSITY

"In medical training, doctors learn to suppress curiosity in order to take rapid, standardized histories," says Jodi Halpern, MD, PhD in an article on Clinical Empathy. [17] The use of electronic health record templates has only made this type of history-taking more impersonal. When we obtain the patient's history by listening to their "own words" with a true interest in hearing their story, we demonstrate true empathy.

Emily Nabors, MD, demonstrates empathy by showing curiosity in her patient's lives: "I try to get an emotional connection with each patient. If I'm able to establish rapport it feels like a friendship."

TRY TO IMAGINE THE PATIENT'S SITUATION

Use whichever cliché you prefer ("walk a mile in their shoes"), but the bottom line is that empathy means trying to imagine the emotions and the situations that your patients are facing. While sometimes this can be relatively straightforward, there are other times when it seems difficult to find an emotion to empathize with. "Even our patients with multiple medical complaints but no real medical problem can garner our empathy – we can feel badly that this is the life that they have chosen as a 'sick person,'" says Dr. Jennifer Keehbauch.

But what happens when we feel that our empathy levels have been crushed out of us? We've just had to give bad news to a patient after being up all night with a sick child, and oh, a hospital administrator just waltzed into the office to discuss those "patient satisfaction" scores. And now we walk into an exam room, not feeling our best, and face a particularly challenging patient.

The reality is that we all have those days, some of us more than others. I surveyed 43 physicians across all specialties with this question: "How often do you have to 'fake' empathy?" Sixty percent (26/43) answered "all the time," although most respondents indicated that they considered the practice of empathy as a deliberate effort, rather than being phony or fake.

"A professional demeanor takes practice and skill – I don't consider that faking. It's part of the job," answered one Family Physician.

One psychiatrist in my survey reflected, "Empathy comes with time – if you are really listening to a person, over time they become likeable, even when things didn't start out that way. When you understand what they have dealt with and why they are in the situation they are in, the empathy just comes – because it is easy to imagine yourself in that position."

Even if we're having one of those days where we just can't drag empathy out of ourselves, we can learn to show it even if we don't truly feel it. Jennifer Keehbauch, MD, Family Physician and Women's Health Fellowship Director, says that practicing empathy will lead to true feelings of empathy: "I firmly believe in the 'fake it 'til you make it' philosophy. I find that if you just fake it until 10 am, you can usually get through even the worst day."

ROCK STAR TIP:

Take an acting class

The trick to showing empathy when you don't really feel it is to be convincing – and this is where acting lessons can help develop the Rock Star persona.

I'm firmly convinced that the most important class I took in preparing to become a physician had nothing to do with the hard sciences. High school drama club taught me more interpersonal technique than anything I learned in my Clinical Skills med school course.

My theory has scientific validity with a study from the American Psychological Association showing that teaching role-playing (or acting) can not only help students to appear empathetic, but can actually create true empathy. Just *acting* empathetic was shown to reduce the "innate empathy associated with the medical school experience."[18] Another study backed this up, finding that people who are naturally introverted are actually happier when they *act*, or pretend, to be extroverted.[19]

Although not an absolute "Rule," participating in a drama club or acting class is invaluable to becoming a Rock Star physician. Let's be realistic for a minute. None of us feel truly empathetic all the time.

As noted in an earlier section, studies show that, as medical students progress through school, empathy levels significantly decline. There are lots of thoughts on why this happens – a defense mechanism to shield the psyche from the pain and suffering all around; the sense of being beaten-down or compassion fatigue; role modeling of more senior students and residents. Regardless of the reasoning, the medical profession has a way of beating the crap out of you. It's no wonder that physicians have high rates of suicide. But the public has no idea about any of this; remember much of what they know comes from the latest episode of "Scrubs" or "Grey's Anatomy."

So, let's take a clue from Hollywood television drama and incorporate a bit of acting into our day-to-day profession, especially since we know that we are on-stage.

Instead of: "I'm not a doctor but I play one on TV," how about: "I'm a doctor who plays a TV doctor."

Listen, I'm no Meryl Streep. The most acting experience I have comes from small-town high school productions of "Fiddler on the Roof" and corny vaudeville skits more than 20 years ago. Doesn't matter. In those small roles, I learned how to portray a character that wasn't me. Like those annoying celebrities on "Inside the Actors Studio," I could ask myself: "Who is this character? What does she think? Why does she do the things she does?"

No one expects you to win an Oscar - just put your own personal feelings and behaviors to the side for a little while and pretend to be someone else – someone caring, someone competent, compassionate; whatever qualities you would want in your own physician. It's not so much "faking it" as it is embodying the characteristics that create a good bedside manner.

So, when you're having a tough day, just before you open the exam room door click your brain into acting mode and *become* a "Rock Star" doctor.

CONVEYING CONFIDENCE

Returning back to our list of patient-desired physician characteristics, let's focus on the quality of confidence. Remember our Rock Star performer? He prances onto the stage in a crazy outfit - skintight leopard leggings, a purple scarf, big '80s blown-out hair, maybe a ridiculous hat, but he *owns* it and, therefore, the fans buy it. Likewise, learning to show confidence is one of the keys to becoming a Rock Star physician.

Here's another definition from the Oxford Dictionary: "Confidence: A feeling of self-assurance arising from one's appreciation of one's own abilities or qualities."

And we really should feel good about our accomplishments. According to the American Academy of Family Physicians (AAFP), the average graduating FP has spent a total of 21,000 hours studying medicine, with 6,000 hours in lectures and self-study in the first two years of medical school, another 6,000 hours in clinical rotations, and 10,000 hours of patient care in residency.[20] Clearly, we have acquired the abilities and qualities of a physician during these years of training.

But despite this massive amount of education and training, we may not *feel* self-assured when we start our own clinical practice. It is easy to feel overwhelmed with the responsibility of patient care and clinical decision making.

Nonetheless, the bottom line is that patients want a confident-appearing doctor. The Rock Star physician has to learn to portray a façade of confidence or self-assurance in our own abilities. At the same time, we must avoid the cockiness that can come from too-much self-assurance.

So, how to convey confidence, even if we may not feel it? We have to act confident. Here's how.

1. **Body language.** A confident physician walks into a room with her head held high. She stands or sits up straight with her shoulders back and chest out. She has a firm handshake. Practice your posture in the mirror or have a friend critique you. Practice shaking hands. Sounds silly, but practicing acting confident will lead to feeling confident.

2. **Eye contact.** Good eye contact is critical to showing confidence. A confident doctor looks at the person to whom he is speaking and not at the computer or chart. This can be especially tough with an electronic health record, but it's essential.

3. **Speech.** Confident doctors do not mumble or talk to the floor. They speak clearly, loudly, and without rushing. Practice your medical "spiel" in the mirror or with a friend.

4. **Attire.** Professional attire, including a white coat, has been shown to inspire patient confidence in physicians.[21] As Dr. Ariel Cole, Rock Star geriatrician, says, "Dress the part."

5. **Attitude.** A confident physician does not make self-deprecating comments or put herself down. He doesn't say things that frighten patients – like "This is the first time I've done this on my own," or "I have no idea what is wrong with you." Not to say that a doctor shouldn't admit when she doesn't have the answer! However, a statement like "I have quite a few thoughts about what is going on, but I want to do some more testing to determine the correct diagnosis" is more reassuring. Also, if you need to look something up, saying something like "The science and guidelines on this topic are constantly evolving. Let's just take a look to make sure that there isn't anything new that has come up in the last few weeks." You look confident and extra-thorough.

6. **Keep studying.** "Thinking back to my first few years in private practice, I realized that while I didn't have the same experience as more seasoned doctors, I *did* have the resources available," says Roberta Chung, MD. "If I didn't know the answer, I would tell the patient: 'This is something I'm going to have to do research on to give you the best care.' They respected and appreciated that I was going the extra mile to make sure I was doing the right thing. I also did lots of extra reading and research to get comfortable with the medical conditions I was managing." Unfortunately, there is no Rock Star secret to hitting those books!

SHOWING YOUR HUMANITY

Patients value humanity – they want to feel that their doctor is like them. As Carlos Portu, MD, board-certified Internist in Naples, Florida and 2012 Physician of the Year for Physicians Regional Health System says, "People want to feel like you're human. They want to be able to connect with you on a certain level so that they feel comfortable talking about things that may be embarrassing."

One of the ways that Dr. Portu shows his humanity is by sharing small details about himself with his patients. "When patients ask me how I'm doing, I try to share something about myself. You don't have to reveal your deepest darkest secrets, but it helps when your patients have a little bit of empathy for the things that we go through. They need to know that things aren't always hunky-dory just because you have an MD behind your name."

Patients like this, especially when shared information pertains to their own situation and is kept brief and relevant to the patient.[22] Doug Meuser, MD, Sports Medicine physician at the University of Central Florida and Family Medicine Faculty of the Year finds sharing personal information with patients helpful. "I do whatever it takes to get the patient engaged in the fact that I really care for them. If the information that I'm going to provide about me is to assist them with their health care, then that is fine." He notes that in the University setting: "Younger people love for me to share what I would tell my daughter; 'if you were my son or daughter, here's what I would tell you.'"

THE PERSONAL TOUCH

Patients report that the ideal doctor has a personal touch, which involves getting to know the patient as a whole, rather than a number or disease process. One way to show a personal touch is to show familiarity with the patient's medical history, family situation or hobbies and interests.

"Take an interest in the social life of your patients," advises Carlos Portu, MD. "If you're not naturally the most happy-go-lucky person, and not everyone is, write yourself a note on some small detail, and try to mention it at the next visit. Try to create a new memento for the next time that you can ask them about. The patient will feel that you took a personal interest in them."

Personal touch means knowing why the patient is in the office before you walk into the room – you can get this by a quick glance through the chart or a word with the nurse before entering the exam room.

"I always ask my MA to remind me of the patient's personal info," says Dr. Jennifer Keehbauch. "If the MA spent five minutes talking about the patient's cruise, I can just breeze in and say – wow – I heard all about your amazing cruise! And the patient transfers the time they spent with the MA onto me."

Studies show that physicians didn't need to recall extensive details to show a personal touch. Just a small detail of importance to the patient is endearing, in particular remembering and asking about a spouse or child.

Finally, a true personal touch creates a bond with patients, such as touching patients on the arm, hand or giving a hug if appropriate. "I always touch my patients, whether I need to do an examination or not," says Emily Nabors, MD.

HONESTY AND FORTHRIGHTNESS

Doctors are generally considered trustworthy. A poll from the Gallup organization showed that 69% of respondents rated medical doctors as having "high or very high" levels of honesty. Interestingly, the trend seems to be increasing, with 47-58% rating in the 1980's and 90's, up to 63-70% in the 2000's.[23]

In my introduction, I alluded to my early experiences as a young doctor, and a sense of sort of "making it up as I went along." As an autonomous clinician, this isn't an option. We need to feel comfortable with acknowledging the unknown – what is not yet understood by science, and what is beyond a doctor's experience or scope or knowledge.

As Dr. Nabors says, "A physician needs to be genuine. I always tell my patients, 'I'm only as good as what you tell me. If a patient doesn't trust me, they won't tell me what I need to know, and I won't be able to diagnose them accurately.'"

Patients want their doctor to be honest and forthright with them, even when the news may not be good. This is particularly important when discussing end-of-life care, as reviewed in a later section.

Many physicians hesitate to tell the complete truth because we fear that the information will be upsetting or hurtful to a patient. Sometimes we ask ourselves: "Will the patient really want to know this? Wouldn't they be happier *not* to know?" It is not unusual for family members to ask us to protect their loved ones from a painful diagnosis, and they may not want the physician to disclose information for the patient's "own good."

Despite our concern for protecting our patients, a number of studies have demonstrated that patients *do* want their physicians to tell them the truth, even when the news is bad.[24]

So, how do we reconcile this conflict? Directly ask your patient: "How much do you want to know about this situation/ disease/ prognosis?" If we're struggling with how much information to share, it's ok to ask the patient's help in the matter.[25]

ROCK STAR TIP:

Directly ask your patient how much information they want to receive

It is our responsibility to provide truthful information so that our patients can make informed decisions about their health. Our goal should be to be as honest and forthright as possible, tempering the painful truths with kindness and compassion.

APOLOGIZING

Another aspect of honesty is being able to apologize when things go wrong. When I was a brand new doctor, I prescribed hormone replacement therapy to a 50-year old woman at her request. I failed to factor in her recent patella fracture, which was immobilized in a cast. A few weeks later, she was admitted to the hospital with a deep vein thrombosis and pulmonary embolus.

When she saw me back in the clinic upon discharge, I immediately realized what I had done and, although it was painful, I explained my error and apologized profusely. I was stunned when she answered, "I know, the doctor in the hospital told me. But I know you didn't mean to." She's still my patient fifteen years later.

The concept of the physician apology has been much discussed in the last few years with conflicting points of view from lawyers, risk managers, and academicians. Each state has its own law regarding physician apologies. Most encourage an expression of sympathy without considering it an admission of liability.[26]

Saying "I'm sorry" isn't necessarily an admission of guilt or wrongdoing, but it shows that you care. Most communication experts suggest that if your natural inclination is to apologize, do so simply and sincerely.

RESPECT

The ideal physician shows respect for her patients, as well as colleagues and coworkers. Unfortunately, as human beings we struggle with subconscious biases. For example, studies show that physicians show less respect for patients with higher BMIs[27] and exhibit more respect for older patients.[28]

Being aware of our own inherent biases can help us to practice deliberate respect. Using empathy – "there but for the grace of God, go I" – can help us to respect others in less fortunate situations. When we feel a sense of revulsion or irritation creeping in, asking ourselves "How would I feel if I were 300 lbs?" or "What would it be like if I was severely hard of hearing or homeless or illiterate?"

While it can be challenging to interact with people who have opinions, philosophies, and religious views contrary to our own, the Rock Star physician knows how to respond noncommittally and redirect the conversation rather than engaging in debate. Practice your generic response: "Politics!" with a wondering expression and little head shake usually works well.

A simple way to show respect is to call our patients by their formal name – title and last name, as appropriate, unless otherwise advised. Using condescending terms like "sweetie" is not respectful.

Maintaining privacy is an essential aspect of respect – keeping our patients appropriately draped when they are disrobed, avoiding discussing patient care where we can be overheard by others, and maintaining confidentiality.

PATIENT ADVOCACY

Although not on the "list" of physician traits, I think that the attribute that ties all of the others together is the concept of becoming the patient advocate. Asking yourself: "Is this in the best interest of my patient?" is the key to providing Rock Star patient care. "Would I do this for myself, my mother, my brother?"

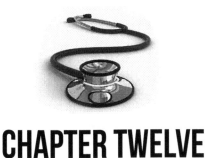

CHAPTER TWELVE

THE ROCK STAR SCENE: SETTING THE STAGE

The Rock Star physician has to have the perfect set, or stage, to work from. While an experienced clinician may already have a well-designed office space, a brand new doc may still be in the planning stage. Either way, the most important element of the Rock Star stage is to set the tone for a positive patient experience.

It is not uncommon for even the most seasoned physician to become immune to the look and feel of the office, as we experience it every day and lose the freshness of seeing it with new eyes. This happened to me a few weeks ago. I stopped into the patient restroom, happened to glance up at the ceiling, and gasped at the thick layer of dust and debris clogging the ventilation duct. Gross! My patients had been staring up at this for years and I had no idea.

Before you, the Rock Star physician, even step onto the stage, your patients have entered on set – in other words, your waiting room.

Make the set as accommodating and pleasant as possible. Most importantly, the waiting room and entire office should be as kept clean as possible. Patients want to think of a medical office as a hygienic environment. Seeing cobwebs and dust bunnies will do little to inspire confidence.

This can be a challenge with a large volume of foot traffic and will require the efforts of the entire office staff to make rounds through the office a few times per day, discarding used Kleenexes, emptying coffee cups, and tossing torn-up magazines.

ROCK STAR TIP:

Engage your staff in regular "rounds" through the office

General cleaning like vacuuming, emptying the trash, and refilling soap dispensers should be happening every day after patients have been seen. Exam room surfaces should be wiped down with anti-viral cleaning solution on a daily basis.

In my current job, I'm lucky enough to have a cleaning service that does a basic cleaning daily. When I worked in an underfunded Federal Health Center, the staff and I drew straws to assign cleaning duties. With everyone working together it wasn't very difficult to maintain a basic level of cleanliness.

As often as possible, a professional deep cleaning is warranted for the more difficult tasks like cleaning baseboards and flooring, touching up paint (it's amazing how quickly wheelchair marks show up on walls), cleaning air ducts, and heavy dusting.

Speaking of dust, follow the recommendations of our allergist colleagues and keep the tchotchkes to a minimum. Anything that doesn't have a purpose is just going to be a source of dust collection. In particular, avoid fake plants! Not only are they dust magnets, but they are tacky. Sorry, but it's true. And as our allergist friends advise, try to avoid carpets, curtains, cushions - all excellent sources of hidden dust and debris.

MINIMIZE GERM EXPOSURE

Your waiting room is a spectacular vector for germ transfer. Look out into your waiting room. Is there someone out there hacking and coughing right next to your well-child visit? If so, plan on seeing that kid back in a week or so with the same illness. Not good.

The Rock Star doctor has her staff trained to quickly remove acutely ill patients from the waiting room into an isolated exam room, or if this is not possible, to ask the patient to wear a disposable face mask. Masks should be available at the front desk with a sign advising potentially contagious people to report their illness to the front staff.

Even better, Emily Nabors, MD, a Family Physician who sees children and adults, suggests "Having a separate sick and well waiting room prevents the spread of illness."

Keep boxes of tissues and hand sanitizer liberally spread throughout the waiting room, as well as trash cans to dispose of waste.

AIR PURIFICATION

After I determined that coming into my office was flaring up my allergies despite massive amounts of antihistamines, I went on a mission to figure out how to clean the air. The Environmental Protection Agency (EPA) recommends that the best way to improve air quality is to allow fresh air to flow through living space by opening windows. This is especially important in energy-efficient buildings which often have poorer indoor air quality.

I would love to open my windows – if only I could. I have never worked in an office with windows that open. Next best option: a fancy air purifier.

I did tons of research into air filters and it was not easy. While I found a lot of material on different options, there was no evidence-based data. Ultimately, I bought a few different products and found my favorite air purifier. Since I bought this filter, I've had patients comment on how fresh the air seems and many requests to find out where I bought it.

Also consider the use of plants for air filtration. Research from NASA in the 1980s showed that some plants are effective at removing formaldehyde and other volatile chemicals from the air. [29] On the flip side, dead or dying plants don't inspire much confidence in a medical office!

Definitely pick a plant that's hard to kill – for me, that's Golden Pothos, the only plant species that I seem to be able to keep alive. Part of the problem, other than not-so-benign neglect, is fluorescent lighting, which, like many humans, seems to be hard on plant health.

An even better option is to hire an office plant service that will care for your plants and replace any that are starting to look unhealthy. Your office will look more attractive and also get the added bonus of psychological benefit that plants provide.

TOP TEN HOUSEPLANT AIR CLEANERS FROM NASA:

1. Areca palm
2. Lady palm
3. Bamboo palm
4. Rubber plant
5. Draceana
6. English Ivy
7. Dwarf date palm
8. Ficus
9. Boston fern
10. Peace lily

MAKE IT COMFORTABLE

When designing your exam room, keep in mind the comfort of your diverse patient population. Many patients will have mobility issues or weight problems. Weaker patients will appreciate the option of a chair with arms. And significantly overweight patients can benefit from larger or armless chairs. It is always heartbreaking to me to see a morbidly obese person jammed into a regular sized chair. That's just another reason why an overweight and sensitive person might hesitate to come to the doctor's office.

"I designed my office to be 'homey," says Ed Douglas, DO, a Rock Star solo physician with Advanced Alternative Healthcare in Springfield, Missouri. "The waiting area is not like most docs' offices. I used home furniture, not typical waiting room furniture. The colors are calming... We get lots of compliments on our office because it isn't a cold, sterile office or hospital feel."

Emily Nabors used spa-like muted earthy tones in her waiting room. "It's like a desert oasis," she says. "I also have windows in the exam rooms to let in natural light."

Temperature control seems to be a particular challenge. It always seems like medical offices are freezing when it's hot outside and stiflingly warm when it's cold out. Try to make sure that the waiting room temperature is kept in a comfortable range. Lighting should be bright enough for comfortable reading. Use side lamps rather than fluorescent overhead lighting if possible. Adding a few table lamps can add a sense of warmth to a standard waiting room.

While aromatherapy plug-ins or air freshener sprays are enjoyed by some patients, be aware that they can create allergic reactions, migraine headaches or even respiratory distress in sensitive patients. My inclination is to avoid these products and use an air purifier system instead (see previous section).

CREATE A CALMING ENVIRONMENT

Oh, how I despise a blaring television in a medical office. That's especially true if the TV is set on any type of news station. No matter what your political preferences, any given news network is likely to offend 50% of your patient population. Not to mention the negative, frightening tone of much television news – of course your patient is going to have high blood pressure by the time they get back into the exam room.

If you absolutely must have a television on in your office, pick a calming channel like a Travel channel or Animal network (puppies and kittens, anyone?). Keep the volume at a reasonable level.

My preference is to skip TV and have quiet music playing, preferably classical or other relaxing music. Nature sounds – soothing ocean surf, for example, is another calming option. "Play peaceful, relaxing music throughout the office and exam/ treatment rooms," says Dr Douglas.

Emily Nabors, MD, also points out that playing music is helpful for "drowning out conversation" and can help with protecting patient privacy.

As mentioned above, the room temperature should be comfortable and lighting appropriate. If you want to get fancy with water features and plants, go for it. Just *no fake plants*!

MAKE IT CONVENIENT

It's always nice when your patients can find your office. While signage can be a major zoning challenge in some communities, do the best you can to make your office easy to see from major roadways. Providing directions when you schedule your initial patient visit is a good idea, as well as sending that information along with new patient paperwork ahead of the office visit.

Do a walk-through of your office building - how difficult is it to wind your way through the building and into your suite? Is the signage adequate to direct patients to your office? Make sure that your office entrance is well-marked and professional appearing.

Inside, the office should have access to an adequately supplied restroom and a water fountain. We find that our patients appreciate a small coffee station - especially for early morning appointments.

Another convenient item is to have Wi-Fi internet access available for your patients. I have found that this is one of the most requested items from my patient population, not only for business people, but for parents with bored children or others who like to pass the time by web surfing.

For your "old-school" patients who still enjoy a good magazine, keep a nice selection of up-to-date reading material to make the wait more palatable. Get a range of magazines for different interests – pop culture, business, fashion, sports, science – anything to keep your patients from getting bored. Keep 'em current - you don't want to be the clichéd doctor with stacks of ancient torn-up issues of National Geographic.

Make sure that some of these magazines make it back to the exam rooms, too – as a patient, there is nothing worse than leaving your reading material in the waiting room only to sit in an exam room with nothing to do. Besides magazines, you may wish to have a few books for browsing - at my office we have a popular "give a book, take a book" rack, which I keep stocked with offerings from the local thrift store.

SETTING THE STAGE – YOUR FRONT DESK

The first person that patients will interact with is your receptionist or front desk "office coordinator." This person is critical to the Rock Star team, as he or she will truly set the stage for the office visit. "Your front desk staff is very, very important," says Dr. Emily Nabors. "They are the doorway to your office."

Roberta Chung, MD, agrees. "The front desk staffer is the first person that your patients see, and the first voice that they hear on the phone. She is almost as important as the office manager, and yet unfortunately in most practices the front desk person is the one making the lowest salary, and with the least investment in the practice. "

The front desk is about as on-stage as you can get. So it's little wonder that front desk staff feel the stress of a medical office. In fact, staff turnover in medical offices is highest among receptionists.[30]

"It's critical to hire the right person, and invest them in their role in growing the practice," advises Dr. Chung. "They need to know that they are an essential part of the team and patient satisfaction."

"Your front staff needs to be someone organized, friendly, and helpful," says Emily Nabors, MD, or have what I call the four 'P's: be Polite, Private, Professional, and Personable.

POLITENESS

Your front staff (as well as the rest of the office staff) should remain polite at all times. This can be difficult (see later chapter on "Dealing with challenging patients"), but is critical to the success of the practice. There is never any excuse for rudeness in a medical office staff. This is an area where the Rock Star physician can provide outstanding role modeling for staff.

Emily Nabors, MD, likes to tell her staff, "We're here to help our patients - We wouldn't be here without them."

PRIVACY

I don't have to tell anyone about the Health Information Privacy and Portability Act (HIPPAA) these days. The whole point of HIPPAA is to ensure adequate privacy in transferring medical records and sharing data with unauthorized users. However, in some facilities, the letter of the law has exceeded the spirit of privacy protection, creating challenges in sharing critical records, and potentially compromising care.

Regardless, the front desk staff must make patient privacy a top priority. Patients should not be able to hear your staff discussing another patient's health information. Data should be shielded from patients standing at the check-in window by positioning computer screens away from probing eyes, and covering any paperwork in sight.

PROFESSIONALISM

The front desk should look professional, as should the people working there. The Rock Star front desk has a polished appearance, with the minimum of posted signs, sticky notes, knick-knacks, or family photos. The counters should be as cleared of debris as possible, keeping charts, manuals, etc. in drawers or cabinets out of sight.

Your front desk staff should be well groomed and professionally dressed. They should appear neutral, essentially blending into the background scenery. Avoid inflammatory hair styles, piercings, etc. It's not a place for personal expression. It's a medical office.

Staff should avoid discussing topics not relevant to the office practice. Talk about last night's date, the latest celebrity gossip or reality show is not appropriate for a patient who may be coming in for a life-or-death situation. It's that good old Golden Rule in action once again.

Try to get your patients out of the waiting area and into an exam room as quickly as possible. When your clinical staff member comes to escort a patient into an exam room, make sure that they call the patient by his or her last name, using the appropriate Mr., Mrs., Dr., etc., unless instructed otherwise. Some patients may actually prefer to be called by their first name - I have an 80-year old patient named Catherine who insists on being called "Kitty," and a nonagenarian named Dolores who must be called "Dolly." However, avoid terms of endearment like "honey," "sweetie," or "dear." They are condescending and inappropriate and only work in the deepest South, if ever.

Make sure that your staff use a friendly tone and avoid terseness. They shouldn't turn their back on the patient – rather, guide the patient with verbal cues, "We're going to turn left at this hallway," "You can leave your purse on this counter while we check your weight," etc. Remember that while the staff member does this a thousand times a day, this may be the patient's first experience.

I also like for my staff members to escort the patients to the check-out area after their appointment is complete. A companionable stroll through the office ends the visit on a positive note, helps the patient to find his way through our office maze, and ensures that a follow-up visit is scheduled.

PERSONABLE

A frequent compliment we get from patients is they feel like family in our office. Patients like to get to know the staff and actually come to care about them, especially our seniors. When one of my nurses had a baby, many patients insisted on seeing pictures and regular updates from me, some even bringing baby gifts!

Your medical team is an extension of you as the Rock Star physician and sets the tone for your own entry onto the scene. Encourage staff to make light small talk while checking vital signs, in a kind and friendly way. Validate and calm any anxieties that the patient may express. Use confident, reassuring tones and a kind voice. Show empathy. Staff members can often learn these qualities from the Rock Star physician role model. So it helps to practice with your staff.

In fact, when I find a lack of experience in patient interaction, I like to role play with my staff so that they can practice in a supportive environment before dealing with real patients. This can be a fun group activity as fellow staff members play patient.

Always address any concerns your patients express about your assistants promptly. Constructive feedback, with kindness, is critical to staff growth and development.

THE ROCK STAR EXAM ROOM

Your examination room should be every bit as clean as your waiting room, if not more. Spend some time sitting in your own exam room. Sit on a chair as well as up on the exam table to gain different vantages. Let your eyes sweep along on the ceiling, above the cabinets, and over the wall equipment as well as the floor. Remove dust-collecting objects, tattered old taped-up signs, and outdated reference material.

Make sure that the temperature in the room is comfortable, table paper from the last patient has been removed, and supplies are organized and out of view as much as possible. The exam room should be designed to protect your patient's privacy. The exam table should not face towards the door. A curtain or screen should be available if patients need to disrobe for an examination.

Rather than use artwork on the walls, I like to have anatomy charts displayed in my exam rooms. What better art for doctor's office than the human body? Charts are inexpensive, interesting for patients to look at, and come in handy when explaining physical features, especially structures like ear, nose, and throat (ENT) and the gastrointestinal system. I keep a chart of the female reproductive system in my gynecology room so that I can point out any areas of concern on the diagram.

There are also wall charts that explain disease processes. I have charts on the pathophysiology of diabetes, heart disease, osteoporosis, and depression. These charts often initiate discussion and questions from patients.

ROCK STAR TIP:

Use wall charts to help patients understand basic anatomy and physiology

MUSCULOSKELETAL CHARTS

Since I have limited wall space and as a family doc I cover the entire body, I use a few different charts in each room. However, in every room I keep a wall chart of the musculoskeletal system.

Why? Because the musculoskeletal system is one of the most common sources of routine medical problems and is often a benign cause of anxiety provoking aches and pains.

Every day I see patients with pain in the back, abdomen or head that they find frightening, but often attributable to muscle strain, sprain or spasm. Naturally, patients presume that the root of the pain is *internal* and immediately worry that the pain in the back is a kidney stone or the pain in the back of the head is a brain tumor.

It is much easier to convince the patient that the pain they are feeling is musculoskeletal when they see a diagram of the extremely complex and inherently interconnected muscle system. "Do you see this big muscle here?" I say, pointing to the psoas major. Once a patient can visualize how the muscles line the back wall of the abdomen, it is much easier to comprehend how pain in the belly or groin can actually be caused by a muscle strain rather than something more sinister.

Even better, says Doug Meuser, MD, Family Physician and Sports Medicine specialist, is to have models of physical structures in the exam rooms. "Patients can point and touch, which gives them a visual and tactile experience. These are great props and really help the patient to understand physical processes."

Much of being a Rock Star doctor is helping patients to understand their body and to reassure them when their symptoms are not caused by a life-threatening ailment.

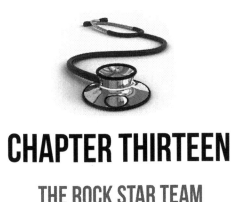

CHAPTER THIRTEEN
THE ROCK STAR TEAM

ROCK STAR CLINICAL STAFF

Most physicians utilize a clinical assistant, usually a Medical Assistant (MA), Licensed Practical Nurse (LPN) or Registered Nurse (RN) to assist with patient care and allow the physician to maximize face-to-face patient time.

Emily Nabors, MD, credits her success to an excellent Registered Nurse (RN), who prescreens every patient chart. "The key to seeing so many patients is to have a RN prep the charts. It's the only way to do volume *plus* quality." This is something that Dr. Ariel Cole has to do herself. "There is no doubt that I could see many more patients if I didn't have to do chart reviews by myself."

But does the nursing training matter in a primary care office? Studies indicate that offices with an RN had higher quality indicator scores and patient satisfaction, as well as improved office efficiency and overall reduced cost of health care[31], with fewer hospital and emergency room visits. [32]

However, other studies have shown improved health outcomes when patient-centered medical homes (PCMHs) utilized medical assistants as the primary clinical team member.[33]

In the real world, many physicians work with less trained clinical staff, mainly Medical Assistants (MA). I polled 45 multispecialty physicians and found that 62% worked with MAs, 22% used Registered Nurses (RNs), and 16% Licensed Practical Nurses (LPNs). Why? Cost-benefit ratio.

According to salary.com, the average clinic medical assistant earns $32,000 per year, while an office LPN makes $40,000, and a RN $62,000. A significant difference, although some physicians feel that the additional cost is worthwhile. Dr. Roberta Chung says, "In an ideal world, an RN has so much more to offer- they can triage patients, provide education, and promote efficiency in an office practice."

So what's the difference in scope of practice?

A medical assistant is not licensed and practices strictly under physician direction. While an MA can perform all of the basic functions of most medical offices, including obtaining vital signs, preparing patients for the physician, and drawing blood work, she cannot assess patients or legally perform triage over the telephone or in person.[34] An added benefit of MA training, on the other hand, can be better knowledge of clerical and billing elements of the medical office.

An LPN completes a year of nursing training; while RNs go on to complete an additional year or more of clinical training. Compared to an MA, an LPN may also perform additional clinical procedures such as starting intravenous lines and inserting Foley catheters. However, compared to a RN, the scope of practice of an LPN is significantly reduced, with restrictions on providing telephone triage or changing the care plan. [35]

While more out-patient physicians tend to hire medical assistants as a way of reducing overhead, Dr. Chung points out that RNs can save physician time. "A good nurse can obtain vital information and give the physician a 'head's up' on psychosocial issues. Once you get the patient's story out, you know the real reason for the visit, and you can really direct your focus and save time. I believe that the additional patient volume that I can see with an RN more than makes up for the difference in nurse salary."

Regardless of which direction is best for your practice, Dr. Keehbauch gives this advice about staff: "Pay them well, train them up, and invest in them as a person. And expect that after you get them 'good' they may leave after 3-5 years."

While many good staff members do leave for other opportunities, keeping staff happy is critical for the success of the Rock Star practice.

Dr. Chung recommends giving positive feedback to staff. "I tell my nurse 'I'm so glad you found that out,' when she gives me helpful details about patients." Doug Meuser, MD, recommends "Try to treat them nicely, understanding that the staff is on-stage sometimes 9-1/2 hours per day."

Staff education is also important. "Do a 'needs assessment,'" says Dr. Meuser. "Find out what they are interested in. Educate your staff when they are interested in being educated, and if I'm good, I can get them interested in what I'm interested in."

I have team meetings every week or two where I include a short review of a clinical topic – such as a new medicine or study, or a topic suggested by the staff.

Spending time with your staff outside of the office can be positive for morale as well. I try to have a staff dinner outside the office for holidays and birthdays. And I also take the team to lunch every month or two as a group.

ROCK STAR TEAMWORK

A former manager used to call my office staff the "Navy Seals" of the organization. Every team member in my office has a role and responsibility, and each and every person is essential to the mission. "A good medical team is one where every team member takes ownership," says Paul Marsolek, a published author on leadership and physician specialist.

The medical team needs to be carefully selected and developed with a physician leader. When new physicians start work in already established practices, they may not have the opportunity to be involved in team selection – this is a big mistake, according to Paul Marsolek. As he says, "Sometimes administrators unknowingly set up new physicians to fail, by providing lesser qualified staff to the newest doctor. The Rock Star doctor needs a Rock Star team. Demand to have a team built around *you.*"

This is especially important when a doctor struggles with what Dr. Jennifer Keehbauch calls the "niceties" of interpersonal relationships. "If you're good at efficiency, but not really a 'people person,' hire an MA that is. I don't like small talk, so I have my staff get the 411 - that way I can just recap what the patient talked with my assistant about, and the patient thinks that I was talking to her longer that I actually was."

The bottom line is that the medical team is there to support the patient-physician relationship, allowing the doctor to maximize face-to-face time and minimize paperwork[36]. As Mr. Marsolek says: "Doctor time is more expensive than staff time."

84

So, how to develop a Rock Star team?

DEFINE ROLES AND RESPONSIBILITIES

Each team member needs to have a defined role and should be performing up to the level of their skills and licensure. It is very important that as many members of the team as possible be cross-trained to perform alternate job responsibilities in the case of an unexpected team member's absence. In our office, we created a staff flow sheet that details every element of a patient encounter in order to ensure consistency with our care and also to serve as a check-list for newer staff members.

Sample: Clinical Assistant Responsibilities in an Adult Routine Visit for Dr. Rock Star

- ✓ Open encounter: "Adult Office Visit"

- ✓ Enter "chief complaint (cc)" **cannot** be "establish" or "follow-up"

- ✓ Review and update/reconcile medication list

- ✓ Does patient need refills? Prepare prescriptions either written or for doctor to ERx.

- ✓ Make sure that the preferred pharmacy information is correct

- ✓ Update allergies

- ✓ Update past medical, surgical, family, and social histories. Make sure that women have OB history (pregnancies/ births) entered into the histories

- ✓ Update health maintenance form

- ✓ Enter vital signs. Always pull forward or enter height so that BMI will calculate. Always update LMP in women of child-bearing age. If there is any chance that a woman is pregnant, inform doctor/ do pregnancy test

85

✓ Review Dr. Rock Star's plan from the last office note. Anticipate and prepare any necessary data such as labs, radiology, specialist notes, etc.

✓ Administer any necessary tests such as UA, pregnancy tests, rapid flu/ strep, etc.

✓ Advise Dr. that patient is ready

Accountability is critical to the Rock Star team. The physician has to trust that his staff is accurate, ethical, and thorough. Any breach of trust must be addressed immediately and ruthlessly before patient care is compromised. Lying, falsifying the medical record, and deliberate breach of confidentiality are grounds for termination.

Empowerment is essential for a Rock Star team. This means that after training the staff, the physician needs to learn to delegate responsibility liberally, and avoid micromanaging. Trust goes both ways – once you trust your team, they need to trust that you won't be changing the rules suddenly or breathing down their neck for small details.

ASSESS THE GROUP DYNAMIC

"Staffing is always the wild card," says Roberta Chung, MD. "Everyone in your office will be qualified, but they may not all get along well together – it's the intangible question of 'do they gel?'" Dr. Chung recommends assessing the group dynamic – "If one person detracts significantly from the group, you may need to reconsider that position. When the staff is happy working together, the patients feel it."

The physician must take a leadership role in developing a Rock Star team. Holding regular meetings, or "huddles," are important to solicit ideas and find out where help and additional resources are needed. Delegate responsibility to your office manager and other staff members whenever possible. Don't get overly involved in conflict negotiation – leave this to your office manager, as dealing with interpersonal relationships can be very time-consuming and draining for the busy physician.

Make sure that your staff has adequate resources to do their job efficiently. Everyone needs their own work space, employing ergonomics as much as possible. As promoters of health, we need to start at home to set a good example. I hate to see staff members getting carpal tunnel syndrome from improper wrist support on the keyboard or neck pain from the telephone, when simple solutions such as wrist pads and headsets can be employed.

Create written processes and protocols to simplify and standardize the systems in your office, with tools and resources readily available. If the staff can easily find information, they won't have to interrupt the physician needlessly. This is especially important for patient care. The team needs to know where to look in your notes and the medical record to find information, answer questions, and arrange follow-up for patients, rather than asking the physician directly every time.

Set your expectations high: Expect good work, attention to detail, and a commitment to the office mission statement of providing patient care. When this is being done, reward your staff. While financial compensation is always welcome, positive feedback is critical. Paul Marsolek, a physician communication specialist, advises "When you hear compliments about your staff, share the good news. Get positive comments out there. Just being associated with positivity improves relationships."

HOW MANY STAFF MEMBERS DO YOU NEED, ANYWAY?

You can do all that "industry benchmark FTE (full-time equivalent)[37]" stuff, but ultimately every physician needs to determine the staffing that is comfortable for her goals and patient population. For example, when I worked in a Federally Qualified Health Center, with extremely low health literacy and very ill patients, I had additional staff members to perform detailed clinical education and assist with referrals to specialists, which could include helping the patients find transportation and providing a translator. We had extra clerical staff as well, as the demands of Medicaid and sliding-scale payment fees created mountains of paperwork, as did efforts to assist patients with financial resources like pharmaceutical assistance programs.

When I joined a corporate hospital employed model, I was surprised to find that I would be assigned only *one* clinical assistant and *one* "secretary." Although I certainly didn't need the volume of staff to work with a more educated and resource-rich population, it wasn't long before my staff couldn't keep up with patient needs and I had to add another clinical staff member and front desk person.

For a busy Family Practice (as in, a Rock Star practice!), at least two clinical assistants are needed to keep the flow moving. The physician should be able to walk out of Exam Room 1, leaving an assistant to help that patient with labs, education, etc, and into Exam Room 2, as your second assistant is preparing a patient in Exam Room 3.

If you are going to use your staff for more responsibilities such as collecting documentation, you may even consider a third clinical staffer. Data entry is one of the most time consuming aspects of the medical record and can create a terrible time burden on the physician. The improvement in quality of life (i.e. not spending hours after work with your computer) may be worth the extra staffing expense.

ROCK STAR TIP:
Offer one-stop shopping for your patients

Having additional staff members can support the one-stop shopping model of health care – providing as many services as possible at the office visit. At my office, we offer phlebotomy for our patients – patients love the convenience and I love knowing that I am going to get my results.

We also run our own Coumadin clinic with point-of-care finger-stick INR testing – no more having to track the patient down after clinic to adjust Coumadin dosing.

Extra staff will also allow you to keep your office open during the lunch hour, a valuable convenience for your patients – how many times have you tried to call the doctor during your lunch break only to get a recording that the office will reopen at 1? The only way to manage this is to have additional staff to "cover" the front.

Finally, having additional staff allows the doctor more flexibility in doing office procedures and more time-consuming care like wound management. The Rock Star physician can waltz into the procedure room, perform the biopsy or ingrown nail removal, and leave the patient in the good hands of the nurse. Dr. Ariel Cole, a Family Physician faculty member, feels the lack of a dedicated nurse especially when she needs to do procedures. "I could be so much more efficient – instead I have to set up all the supplies myself, which takes longer."

And now, what you've all been waiting for…

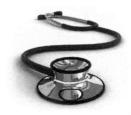

CHAPTER FOURTEEN

THE ROCK STAR DEBUT – GETTING "ON-STAGE"

The stage is set and ready for our star to make his appearance. As you stand in the wings (or outside the door), prepare to transform into Rock Star physician. As Doug Meuser, MD, says, "When you open the door, you're walking on stage." The best way to begin this transformation is to prepare yourself for a positive experience, starting with a smile.

A common positive response on my patient satisfaction surveys refers to smiling both by the physician and the staff. In general, people like a smiling face. And a friendly smile starts the office visit on a positive note. Believe it or not, even when anticipating bad news, patients prefer a smile to a dour expression.

It sounds funny, but you may need to practice smiling. Sometimes it's easy to bring a smile to your face, but other times smiling is the last thing that you feel like doing. You're running an hour behind, you're distracted with personal issues, your patient is scowling at you as you walk in the door; there are probably multiple reasons that you just want to get the day over with. Your natural facial expression may likely be annoyance, frustration, irritability or even downright anger. But you can't show that! Remember… you're on-stage.

Take a deep breath. From the minute your hand is on the outside doorknob, before you even open the door, big smile, and turn on the charm. You don't have to mean it. Although *sometimes* when you start smiling, you may feel just a little happier. Maybe not, but actually feeling happy is not mandatory. You just have to fake it for the next 10 seconds or so. You can do it.

"Knock-knock." I always tap and call-out as I open the door. Immediate eye contact, big smile like this is an old friend that I am delighted to see. I'm wearing professional business attire, my ID tag labeling me as a "Physician" is clearly showing, and of course, I've got the good old Littmann stethoscope draped around my neck. I choose not to wear a white coat in my office setting where most of my patients are established and know me well by sight. Although I do wear one when I round in the hospital or other medical facilities as a form of quick identification for hospital staff and patients.

THE GREAT WHITE COAT DEBATE

Studies are mixed on patient preference for the "White Coat." While some studies indicate that patients prefer to see their doctor dressed in a white coat, identification badge, and a tie for men[38], other studies support a preference for semiformal attire, preferably with below-the-elbow attire[39]. On the other hand, another study shows that patients had *no* consistent preference for their physician's attire. [40]

There is recent concern in the literature over the white coat and tie being a vector for microbes – probably because they aren't washed with anywhere near the regularity of usual attire.

I personally hate wearing a white coat, simply because of comfort. I have never found a classic white coat that fits me comfortably; the fabric is scratchy, it gets caught on things, and it always seems to weigh me down and cause my shoulders to ache.

In medical school and residency, the white coat was of great use – I remember stuffing the pockets with guidebooks, pens, my beeper, a stethoscope, pocket references, and patient notes.

In the out-patient clinical setting, however, I find the white coat unnecessary other than as a means of identifying yourself as "the physician."

In residency, I always admired the attending physicians (usually surgeons for some reason) who showed up for rounds in a suit and tie, sans white coat. Their attire and demeanor seemed to indicate that their self-confidence was more than adequate to prove themselves as "Physician," and no other signal was necessary.

Not that I think that a designer suit is a requirement to be a Rock Star doctor. Any clean, unwrinkled professional business attire shows respect for yourself and for your patient. Below-the-elbow attire seemed to be generally preferred in most studies, always an identification badge, and a smile.

White coat optional.

THE GREAT SCRUB DEBATE

As with the white coat, patients were conflicted about physicians wearing scrubs in the clinic setting. I prefer not to wear scrubs in the office mostly because they never fit correctly – either too long, too big or too small and therefore, horribly figure-unflattering. Even worse, they often wrinkle and look like cheap pajamas.

And just FYI, 79% of unwashed hospital scrubs were found in a study to test positive for gram-positive cocci, some of which was methicillin resistant staph aureus (MRSA). And while hospital-cleaned scrubs are nearly sterile, 44% of bacteria remain on scrub fabric after washing them at home. [41]

While there is no definite evidence that wearing scrubs outside the hospital transmits said bacteria, it can send a negative impression to the public and appear unprofessional.

My opinion: wearing scrubs outside the hospital at dinner, shopping, etc is gross and pretentious ("Look at me! I'm a doctor!").

BACK TO OUR ROCK STAR DEBUT...

Before entering the exam room, the Rock Star doc checks the chart, so that she can personally greet the patient by name, "Mrs. Jones! How *are* you? So good to see you!" And almost always, "So sorry to have kept you waiting!"

Studies show that patients appreciate an acknowledgment that their time is important and are more understanding of late visits when an apology is offered for wait times. I just make the apology a standard part of my greeting, and sometimes I get pleasantly surprised: "Oh, I wasn't waiting long at all!"

Next, the "personal touch" – a nice firm, warm handshake, good eye contact, and then sit in a very relaxed, casual manner. Don't even *think* of looking at the computer yet.

THE "SMALL TALK"

So, here we are with our patient in the exam room. You're still beaming broadly, leaning back in your chair like you're settling in for a long, cozy chat. So begins the small talk. Sounds minor, but this introduction will set the tone for the visit and is a Rock Star secret for making patients *feel* that you spent more time with them.

For my established patients in for a routine visit I like to use: "So, what's new and exciting in your life?" I don't know why that expression became my "go-to" opener, but I've experimented with alternate ice-breakers ("What's going on?," "How may I help you today?," "How has your health been?") and I keep coming back to the "new and exciting" question. Dr. Roberta Chung uses the same opener. "I like to start out on a positive note, because it won't be long before we get to the negatives."

POSSIBLE ROCK STAR DOCTOR OPENERS

"What's new and exciting in your life?"

"I'm glad you're here."

"So good to see you today!"

"And who do you have with you today?" (Shaking hands with everyone in the room)

"What can I do for you today?"

"I'm sorry to hear you're not feeling very well today."

"How has your health been since the last time I saw you?"

"Good morning! And how are you today?"

"Hi, I'm Dr. X, what should we talk about today?"

"Tell me something good today!"

"So what are you doing for fun these days?"

"What's on the agenda?

As previously mentioned, the Rock Star physician will have already glanced at the patient chart (or pre-printed last office note) before entering the room, so we already have a basic idea of why the patient is here.

ROCK STAR TIP:

Check the patient chart before walking into the room

Hopefully, you made a little note in the chart (ideally on the problem list, see later section) of a patient interest, hobby or other detail that can serve as an easy segue into the main topic. "And how is Jenny doing at college? She's majoring in… what again?" Even better if you can find a mutual topic of conversation – "How was that trip to India? I'm thinking of planning that down the road." Remember, we are building our rapport of "pleasant ease and friendliness" before we get down to business. Finding mutual interests is an especially good way of breaking the ice with your more emotionally challenging patients. And when your patients believe that you care about them (remember all that stuff about empathy?), you will get better outcomes.

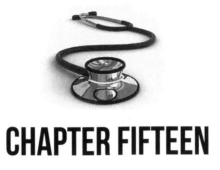

CHAPTER FIFTEEN

LISTENING OR 'SIX SECONDS TO ROCK STAR"

ROCK STAR RULE #5:

Listen to your patients

SETTING THE STAGE FOR ACTIVE LISTENING

One of the most surprising comments that my patient satisfaction surveys return is: "She always listens." At first I was disappointed; listening? That's nothing! Why don't they say: "She always helps me," or "She saved my life?" However, I soon learned that listening is one of the most important and valued qualities that the Rock Star physician can cultivate.

What we did *not* learn in medical school was that many patients don't come to their doctor looking for answers – sometimes they just want to be listened to. This realization can be surprising and disconcerting to many physicians, especially in our early career stage.

ROCK STAR TIP:

Sometimes patients don't want answers; they just want to be listened to

When I first realized that many of my patients weren't coming to me for solutions, my first feeling was annoyance and frustration. Why did I spend all these years in school? Why do they keep coming back to me when they never do any of the things that I advise them to do?

But once I made the connection that simply talking to me made the patient feel better, it revolutionized my practice style from "problem solver" to "Rock Star." It helped me to learn to relax and not try so hard to fix my patient's problems, which in turn lowered my stress level and made me a happier doctor.

Of course, listening is the key to diagnosing medical disease and finding the right treatment. As Emily Nabors, MD, puts it: "If you listen to the patient, they will usually tell you what's wrong with them."

To demonstrate to our patient that we are listening, we need to use certain types of body language and verbal cues which express care and concern -- called active listening. Active listening helps the Rock Star doctor stimulate conversation and gets a nervous patent to open up with his concerns. It helps to overcome barriers of vulnerability, fear, and anxiety, while encouraging patients to tell us the information that we really need in order to help them. Active listening is a key to Rock Star success, and it can be learned.

CHARACTERISTICS OF ACTIVE LISTENING[42]

Use of "active listening responses" like "uh huh," "oh," "all right," "I see," "Hmm."

Eye contact

Sit down, preferably at eye level

Smile

Giving full attention

Verbal or body expressions of empathy (head shaking, facial expressions)

Personal touch

Sometimes the hardest part of active listening is to learn to force ourselves not to interrupt our patients. This is a particularly challenging issue for the new medical school graduate. After all, we spent much of our educational years trying to be the first one with our hand up to answer the teacher's questions - "Pick me, pick me! I know the answer!"

We come out of medical school trying to be Sherlock Holmes – looking for those little clues that we have been trained to find, in order to make the correct diagnosis, find those zebras and impress your peers with your aptitude. Guess what? You may make an incredible diagnosis, earning you bragging rights amongst your colleagues, but your patient may walk away unimpressed. Why? Because they didn't feel that you listened to them.

THE IMPORTANCE OF SIX SECONDS

Studies show that the average doctor listens for about 18-23 seconds before interrupting patients[43]. And while 23 seconds may seem short for the patient, it can seem an absolute eternity for the busy physician, especially when the first few words seem to be a huge neon-light pointing to the diagnosis ("I've been having this bad pain in my right lower belly…"), or when the opening sentences start out on a rambling tangential soliloquy ("About 15 years ago my second cousin's girlfriend had the same thing...").

Oh, how hard it is to listen attentively, nodding your head sympathetically when the diagnosis is right there or when you want to redirect your patient to *get to the point!*

But the Rock Star doctor knows that it is *critical* to suppress those interrupting urges, for at least a few seconds, until the patient stops talking. Although it may seem an eternity, patients actually finish listing their chief complaint in an average of 29 seconds, only six additional seconds, if they are not interrupted.[44]

SIX SECONDS PER PATIENT, TO GO FROM POOR BEDSIDE MANNER TO ROCK STAR!

As Dr. Ed Douglas says, "I find that if I let most patients go, they tell me almost everything I need to know in 2-3 minutes. They get it all out and they like that because they feel like they have been heard."

Besides improving your patient satisfaction scores, there are other legitimate benefits to waiting those additional six seconds. First of all, given the chance, patients will often tell you what is wrong with them, saving you a lot of investigative work. In fact, one of the best questions that a Rock Star doc knows to ask his patient is "What do *you* think is wrong with you?" Yes, sometimes you'll get a strange look or snarky remark, but more often you will get an insightful and sometimes correct diagnosis.

This is also an opportunity to find out what's *really* on the patient's mind, since patients aren't always completely forthcoming about their concerns. Every doctor has those stories of spending an entire visit on the patient's chief complaint, only to hear that dreaded "…by the way…"

just as you put your hand on the doorknob to leave. Listening also helps you understand the patient's agenda – maybe instead of looking for a treatment or medication, she just needs to hear that her headaches are *not* caused by a brain tumor, so she can stop worrying.

A Rock Star doctor remembers that patients are *not* test-writers. Unlike board examinations, patients don't feed data to evoke the correct multiple-choice answer (if only!). Gathering and correctly interpreting data to form an accurate diagnosis is what separates physicians from other members of the health care team, and the ability to quickly and efficiently obtain relevant information is what makes a doctor a Rock Star. *The extra six seconds may make all the difference.*

SETTING THE STAGE FOR ACTIVE LISTENING

Before you can begin to listen actively to your patient, however, you need to continue to set the stage for a positive experience. While some patients are all-too-willing to spill their life story without any encouragement, many others are afraid to open up, especially at their first visit to a new physician.

SIT AT EYE LEVEL

All doctors should have the experience of sitting in the patient's chair (or on the exam table) – even if it's just for a wellness visit. It's incredible how quickly this role reversal can create a sense of vulnerability, particularly if you are sitting in a cold room dressed in only a paper gown!

As previously discussed, setting the stage involves creating a positive impression from the moment that the physician enters the exam room (and even before).

First, the patient should not be undressed before meeting the physician and ideally should be seated on equal footing. This means having the patient sit in a chair rather than perched up on an exam table and with the doctor also seated rather than hovering above. If you must have the patient on an exam table, at least make sure that the back is up so that they can comfortably lean back – especially important for seniors or those with back issues.

EYE CONTACT

It's so easy, but for some reason many docs struggle with the ability to create good and useful eye contact. No, we're not talking about a staring contest. Just a connection between the eyes that says, "I'm focusing on you and nothing else." At least for the next 29 seconds.

Eye contact is not just a cool psychological trick that the Rock Star doctor can use to engage the patient, although it certainly is critical to show care, concern, and confidence. It is as useful for the diagnostician as it is to bedside manner. A well-trained physician will obtain a wealth of clinical information within those first few seconds of eye contract. The eyes express emotion – pain, happiness, apprehension – when the rest of the body may not.

So stop looking at the chart or your computer, and look your patient in the eyes.

PERSONAL TOUCH – THE HANDSHAKE

As you engage in eye contact, smiling of course, the Rock Star doctor will reach out for a warm handshake, creating the small bond of personal touch. Personal touch shows the patient that the doctor is "on their level" rather than above them, which sets the stage for a useful give-and-take conversation.

With certain cultural groups, there may be alternate greetings. For example, in Mexican-American culture, a handclasp simultaneously with an air-kiss is considered a much warmer greeting than a handshake alone. The Rock Star physician will find out the acceptable cultural nuances of the patient populations he works with and use those to his advantage in appearing oh-so-affable.

Ladies: Beware of the powerful male handshake. Don't wear a right hand ring unless you want to crush your fingers to the bone. I like to extend my hand fairly straight to avoid a real grip, and use my left hand to kind of clasp the recipient's hand. Another option is to shake the patient's wrist, again, using the left hand in a clasp to show warmth.

Docs, the hand "bump" a la Howie Mandel is *not* affable. If you are so OCD that you can't shake your patients' hands, seek a psychiatrist or consider a non-direct patient contact specialty.

BODY LANGUAGE

I love those tabloid magazine articles where a body language expert takes photos of celebrities together and interprets their emotions. While I'm not sure that photographs, snapshots in time, can tell the whole story, the Rock Star doctor knows that understanding body language is essential in both creating the caring physician persona as well as interpreting patient cues.

One of the most challenging aspects of body language in this era of computerized medical records is avoiding the temptation to engage more with the computer than with the patient. This is tough – documentation is so essential to getting paid for your medical care that physicians are often forced to spend more time with their computer than with their patients.

An essential aspect of positive body language is to avoid staring at the computer as much as possible. If you must keep your attention on the computer in order to review information, let the patient know what you are looking for, frequently turning your head to look at the patient, and swinging the screen so that they can see what you are doing. They probably can't make heads or tails of it, nor read the tiny writing (after all, *you* barely can), but at least they're engaging in a shared experience with you.

INCORPORATING THE ELECTRONIC HEALTH RECORD ON-STAGE

Upon entering the room after knocking, the Rock Star physician greets her patient with a smile, a friendly greeting, and a warm handshake. She sits on the same level as the patient, in a relaxed posture as if she has all the time in the world and there is nowhere else she would rather be (see section on "Take an acting class"). She maintains eye contact and totally ignores the elephant in the room – the Electronic Health Record – at least for the first few moments. "I need to act like the patient is the most important object in the room, not me, and not the EHR," says Doug Meuser, MD.

Once the stage is successfully set in this positive way, the physician can make small talk while she goes through the mundane chores of logging into the computer, clicking however-million boxes to open the medical record, and otherwise organizing the documenting aspect of the visit. At this point, she will have to acknowledge the necessary evils of the computer intrusion into the visit - one of the biggest challenges to active listening. It's so much easier to nod and empathize while scribbling in a chart, as compared to clicking between computer screens!

We'll talk in a later section how the Rock Star doctor learns to use the EHR in an efficient and less painful manner, keeping it out of the patient-physician experience as much as possible.

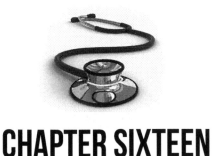

CHAPTER SIXTEEN
EMPATHY AND DEMONSTRATING INTEREST

So to recap, body language tells the patient either:

1. I am interested in what you have to say and I want to help you or:

2. Let's get this over with

Although you may be feeling the latter, you *must* learn to portray the former.

The best way to show interest is to sit down. Repeat after me: Standing = BAD. Sitting = GOOD. Ideally, you'll be sitting at the same level as the patient, all the easier to give good eye contact.

Try to sit facing the patient, although depending on your computer positioning, this might be very difficult. Office architects seem to be more interested in where the electrical outlets are rather than the positioning of physician to patient. Some offices require the physician to turn his back completely to the patient in order to document – a true crime!

Good body language may involve turning completely away from the computer (gasp!) but better to turn your back on an inanimate object than your practice's life-blood. After you develop an acceptable level of rapport, most patients will tolerate physician attention to the computer, at least for a certain amount of time before they get restless.

The Rock Star doctor acts as if he has nothing better to do in the world than to be sitting with this patient, right now, for as long as it takes. Of course, this isn't true, but with the correct body language, this will *seem* to be the case.

The right body language will also make your patient feel that he has spent more time with you than he actually has – many patients refer to my "thoroughness" during the office visit – when in actuality they aren't getting more than the usual 10-15 minutes. It just *seems* thorough because all attention is on them during that time period.

In fact, the actual length of an office visit is *not* significantly correlated with higher patient satisfaction. Rather, it is the perception of time spent that is most important.[45] That's great to know in a busy medical office!

DEMONSTRATE INTEREST

We've talked earlier about how important empathy is in the medical encounter and how demonstrating interest is a great way to show empathy. But how do we achieve the impression of complete interest? Once comfortably seated, facing the patient, maintaining good eye contact, the Rock Star doctor leans back a little with an expression of interest on his face, as if he is sitting down with a good friend for a friendly chat. He makes a little small talk – holidays, travel plans, weather, "How's the family?" – whatever. He knows better than to talk religion or politics, unless perhaps, he is very well-versed in the patient's beliefs and agrees with them! If the patient brings up a controversial subject, the Rock Star doc makes empathetic head movements and noncommittal responses that are open to interpretation – most patients will assume that you are agreeing with them, which is probably fine. You're not running for political office any time soon, are you?

When the patient speaks, the physician leans in a little, showing interest in hearing every word. Nodding, tongue clucking, head shaking, "no kidding!," "really?," and other forms of response are useful for demonstrating interest and listening. Prepare a few noncommittal responses ahead of time – it's doubtful you're truly interested in Aunt Sally's recent hemorrhoid surgery outcome, but you sure can act like you are!

The Rock Star doctor allows *no* interruptions into the examination room while in with the patient, other than in emergencies – the staff should know this and be well trained. That means *no* cell phones, watch checking or answering messages on the computer during the office visit. Sounds obvious, but it's amazing how many patients of mine complain that the doctor actually answered a cell phone during their visit!

So, you're sitting down, you've made a little small talk, you're engaging with the patient - it's time to get down to business. You've used up about 60-90 seconds. Now you're ready for the patient's uninterrupted 29 seconds, all eye contact and interested body language. Let's get into the nitty-gritty: "So what brings you in today?

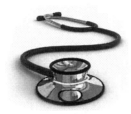

CHAPTER SEVENTEEN

ESTABLISH AND DEVELOP THE PATIENT'S AGENDA

The first step in establishing the patient's agenda is ascertaining his or her goals. The patient's agenda is the most important aspect of the physician office visit and acknowledging the patient agenda is the key to communication success.[46]

That doesn't mean that you are going to spend the bulk of the office visit focusing on the patient's agenda! It just means that you need to *listen* and hear what they have to say before you dive into *your* agenda as a physician.

A way to establish the patient's agenda after listening is to repeat and clarify your understanding of the patient's concern. "So what I hear you saying is… is that right?"

This technique will prevent misunderstandings and save time. It will also help you to explore the patient's fears and concerns, encouraging them to open up to you. As Dr. Emily Nabors says, "If patients don't trust me, they won't tell me what I need to know, and I won't be able to make the correct diagnosis." She likes to tell her patients, "I'm only as good as what you will tell me. Tell me as much as you can so that I can do a better job."

ENCOURAGE WRITTEN LISTS

While some doctors cringe when they see patients clutching a long handwritten list of issues, the Rock Star doctor knows that lists are a great way of homing in on the important issues and keeping patients focused. I love it when my patients bring me written questions and concerns, because it saves me time in trying to drag the history out of the patient and helps me to gauge their understanding of health issues.

"It makes me crazy to wait for a patient to think of that one last thing… 'Wait a minute, it will come to me!' I don't have the next five minutes to wait for you to think about it. Make a list!" says Dr. Ariel Cole, Geriatrician. "It's much faster for me to look their list over so that I can at least acknowledge their concerns."

When reviewing the patient's written list of concerns, I usually take the paper from the patient and we read through it quickly together. Simple responses (they often are!) can be marked on the paper, and issues that are better addressed at a later visit can be denoted. I like to keep a copy of the list with my responses for my file, which then incorporates into the office note – less typing for me!

I also don't mind when patients bring in information gleaned from the Internet, magazine articles or the newspaper. Patients are often hesitant to tell me about their research ("I know you doctors hate this…") but I never criticize independent research. Instead, I encourage my patients to allow me as their trusted physician to interpret the finding, explaining that not all resources have the same reliability. Sometimes the patient's research will actually teach *me* something, although more often I am dispelling misconceptions or unrealistic treatment promises ("no, unfortunately there is nothing available that will make you lose 20 pounds in a week" – as if I would hide that from my patients!)

SHOW CONCERN

It is not uncommon for patients to be afraid to open up to their physician. Being a patient is a position of great vulnerability--in particular if they have had a bad previous experience in the health care system, are anxious about what the doctor might tell them or feel that they may be judged negatively. Encourage and validate the patient's opportunity to talk. Signs of patient anxiety include statements like, "I don't want to take up much time, I know you're busy," or "I know you have other/sicker patients waiting…"

Be sure to emphasize that the patient is the most important person to you at that moment. This means no interruptions from outside the exam room except for emergencies – your staff should know this. The patient gets your full and complete attention. Over time, this validation will usually gain even the most apprehensive patient's trust.

Remember, many patients don't *want* their problems solved! There may simply not be a solution or the options are not viable – or the patient simply isn't ready. While sometimes it's obvious that your patient is just looking for a listening ear, other times it may take multiple visits of them rejecting your suggestions or not following through with treatment plans before you get the idea. But once you make the connection, life suddenly gets a lot easier. Instead of putting on your thinking cap and scrolling through the patient's chart as she starts to report her symptoms, you can turn away from the computer, fold your hands on your lap, and settle into "listening" mode.

So settle in, set your internal alarm clock (hey, we're not on the psychiatry one-hour model, after all!), and practice your best listening affect.

DEVELOPING THE PHYSICIAN AGENDA

You've listened quietly until the patient has finished her introductory statements, you have clarified your understanding of her concerns and goals, and now you're ready to develop *your* medical agenda. Here is where your medical training finally comes into play and you can enter into diagnostician and problem solving mode. The Rock Star doctor can start delving into the details, inquiring into the history more deeply with probing questions. At this point, it's ok to start redirecting the patient back to the issue at hand if they get off track. This is also where you will start to manage the patient's chronic medical issues.

"I always review the patient's information before I enter the room, that way I'm emotionally prepared," says Dr. Ariel Cole. "I've reviewed the CT scan, and there's a big tumor in there. I can't do that in front of the patient, I have to know that in advance. Or maybe the A1c went from 7 to 9 – my agenda just changed. I don't want to find that out in the room."

The challenge in primary care is balancing the concerns of the patient (chief complaint or complaints) with management of chronic medical issues and preventive care. One of the most efficient ways to develop the physician agenda is to utilize the Problem List to organize your thinking. In fact, the Problem List is the Rock Star physician's best friend.

ROCK STAR RULE #6:

Make the Problem List your best friend

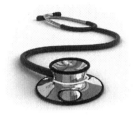

CHAPTER EIGHTEEN

USING A PROBLEM LIST TO DEVELOP THE PHYSICIAN AGENDA

Oh, how hard it is to be a primary care doctor! Not only do we have to treat acute complaints, but we are responsible for staying on top of multiple chronic diseases, following up on abnormal test results, and updating health maintenance at every visit (or so sayeth my residency professors).

In the "olden days," a sheet of paper on the front of the chart would suffice to list all of the patient's chronic problems – diabetes, hypertension, abnormal pap test – probably with space to enter due dates or the date on which each were addressed. A quick look would assure the doctor that nothing important was being missed.

Not so in the average EHR. If you're lucky enough to even have a problem list area, it may be buried within the record or in a place of lower prominence – after all, the bean counters are far more interested in the alphabet soup of PQRS and other "quality health measures." The heck with what the physician needs to care for his patient!

The Rock Star physician will *find* a spot for the problem list and make a point of using it religiously to document issues that require ongoing follow-up. Why? Because it is much simpler for your brain to look at a list in one place, rather than to click through multiple screens and trying to remember what needs to be followed-up on. In fact, managing patient care without a problem list is inefficient, unrealistic, and can be downright dangerous!

"My advice is to keep a very good problem list," says Dr. Doug Meuser. "You've got to do it so that you can actually begin to understand what's important to you and what's critical to patient care."

As David Voran, MD, Family Physician from Platte City, Missouri, says, "No pathologist, radiologist or any other specialist or subspecialist I've seen will touch a problem list. They all say that's your 'problem.' I certainly think it may even be the foundation for the salvation of primary care medicine for us to do so...I rail against the residents I teach who ignore the problem list because 'it's inaccurate' and then blindly exacerbate the situation by not taking the time to review, update and maintain it with the patients."

TRICKS AND TIPS FOR PROBLEM LISTS – MANAGING CHRONIC CONDITIONS

The Problem List is an ever-changing, evolving tool with tremendous versatility. In addition to noting chronic issues – diabetes, hypertension, etc. – it can be used to remark upon those chronic conditions in more detail to provide patient-specific information. For example, rather than your problem list looking like:

DIABETES MELLITUS, UNCONTROLLED (as the EMR is likely to make it show up)

You can addend it to say: Diabetes Mellitus, Type II. Or, because your EHR probably has a character limit, simplify to: DM2.

Now add useful detail: DM2, A1c 6.7 (3/14)

That's a minor change, but one that gives you *so* much more information. What is "uncontrolled" after all? Maybe you use the definition of a Hemoglobin A1c > 6.5. Calling diabetes uncontrolled in the problem list could mean an A1c of 6.7 or an A1c of 12 – a difference with huge clinical relevance. Being more specific in the problem list adds critical information in a small amount of space.

The problem list can also reflect detail such as change over time. For example: DM2, A1c 6.7 (3/14) → 9.2 (6/14).

This is the type of information that a Rock Star physician needs to quickly and efficiently assess multiple problems in one sweep. You can add as much information as the system will allow; often there is a character limit, so the use of your preferred abbreviations will be necessary and helpful. Remove any unnecessary data. Keep the list succinct and uncluttered with irrelevant information.

JUSTIFY MEDICAL DECISION-MAKING

You can also use the problem list to justify or explain aspects of the patient care. This is a good place to look for your documentation on why a patient isn't meeting certain goals so that you don't have to rifle through pages of old notes.

For example, you may have taken your diabetic patient off of her ACE-inhibitor medication because it caused her blood pressure to drop too low. On your problem list you might note: "Hypotension with ACEI."

Having this information readily accessible will quickly satisfy auditors or reviewers – and is especially handy when you get those "Care Consideration" letters from insurance companies: "Dear Dr. Rock Star: From our claims data, we have identified that your patient Jane Doe has diabetes but has not filled a prescription for an ACE-inhibitor. Please consider prescribing an ACE-inhibitor for your patient."

You pull up your patient's chart and, indeed, no ACE-inhibitor is listed on her medication list. Hmm. You're a Rock Star physician, so there must be some good reason why you neglected to start this recommended medication. And sure enough! There, listed right on your Problem List is a reasonable explanation for what the insurance company is questioning as a potential lapse in your medical care.

The Problem List is also a great place to document a patient's decision not to follow your treatment recommendations: "Rectal bleeding - adamantly refuses colonoscopy" for the patient who declines evaluation despite being counseled numerous times.

QUICKLY REVIEW IMPORTANT LAB RESULTS

The problem list is a good place to document recent lab results. Rather than shuffling through lab screens which are often PDF scanned files, jot the results into the problem list. If your system requires you to enter a diagnostic code, as many EHR problem lists do, I like to use V76.62 ("Routine physical lab") and then substitute in the relevant info.

Obviously the problem list isn't made for documenting all of the patient's lab findings, but it will often accommodate a summary of the most important results and dates. This will allow the physician to see basic trends in one place rather than having to create graphs and reports in other parts of the chart that may be more burdensome to use.

NOTE NAMES OF CONSULTANTS AND SPECIALISTS

I also keep details on patient specialists in the problem list. In fact, this will help you meet documentation requirements for your Medicare Wellness visits, which mandate a listing and review of patient problems and specialists – if the info is already noted in the problem list, no additional work required.

Not to mention that if you include details like phone or fax numbers, it is quick and easy to reach out to your consultants without having to shuffle through the medical chart or search the internet for a phone number.

TRACKING PREVENTIVE CARE

The problem list is an ideal place to keep track of due dates to follow up on tests and routine health maintenance. Again, back in the good old days of paper charting, a flow sheet on the front of the chart would show a snapshot of what was due and when. No more. If you're lucky enough to have a functional health maintenance screen on your EMR, it may not be able to be personalized. Or in the case of my system, it may be completely out of date with current guidelines and recommendations (um, that's supposed to be fixed in one of the future upgrades…).

A decent work-around is to utilize the problem list as a common site for listing what tests are due and when. It can also be helpful to add which lab or radiology site the patient uses.

So for example, using the code for "793.80 ABNORMAL SCREENING MAMMOGRAM," you can convert into your own medical shorthand: "Abnl mmg, f/u views due 2/2016." Or "COLON POLYPS" can become "Polyps, colonoscopy due 5/18, Dr. Smith."

I also like to list the date of the last Wellness Visit to stay on top of my annual coding – this way the Rock Star doctor won't miss out on annual preventive visits, now covered for patients at 100% for Medicare and for most commercial insurances--and is well-reimbursed.

ACCESS INFORMATION FOR A PERSONAL TOUCH

The Rock Star physician uses the Problem List as a source of personal information on her patient. Again, back in the "olden days," docs used to jot small details on the margins of the notes – something personal about the patient that can help to strengthen the patient-physician relationship. "Daughter Mary just left for college." "Dog had puppies." "Loves to golf." What better intro to a patient visit than starting off on a personal note: "So how's the golf game?" or "Have those puppies destroyed your house yet?"

Now that we lack margins for scribbling notes, the Problem List can be a useful place to store nuggets of information. You can also make notes to yourself about things to remember about the patient – "Dr. Jones' mother" – "daughter has cancer" – to ensure sensitivity.

A caveat to the use of personal information is to keep in mind that the problem list is a part of the medical record – although continually alterable, the list usually prints out in patient notes. Be sure to keep the data as professional and objective as possible, naturally avoiding any type of inflammatory remarks – "noncompliant," "always late." You get the picture. The Rock Star physician should control the problem list. I don't like other staff members to alter the information – this way I feel confident of the accuracy.

Ultimately, whatever is important for your patient care should go into the problem list, in the easiest way that you can understand and that works within the constraints of your particular EHR.

THE PROBLEM LIST FORM

ORDINARY PROBLEM LIST	ROCK STAR PROBLEM LIST
DMII W/O MENTION OF COMPLICATIONS	DM2, A1c 7.3 (3/14) → 6 (6/14), ophth Dr Jones, foot exam 3/14
HYPERLIPIDEMIA NEC/NOS	Hyperlipidemia, intolerant of all statins
AB MAMMOGRAM NOS	Abnormal MMG, due to recheck 2/14 (XYZ Radiology)
ABDOMEN/PELVIS SYMP NEC	Chonic abd pain, GI w/u/CT normal 5/12
ABN FUNCTION STUDY NEC	Elev LFTs, recheck normal (2/12)
ADJUST DIS W ANXIETY/DEP	Situational anxiety (husband ill with cancer)
ABN CNS FUNCT STUDY NEC	MRI brain – small vessel disease (9/10)
VASCULAR DEMENTIA,UNCOMP	Mild dementia, MMSE 27/30 (1/11) → 26/30 (2/14)
CRBL ART OC NOS WO INFRC	Hx TIA 2004
GENERAL MEDICAL EXAM	Wellness visit done 8/10/14
SCRN UNSPCF VIRAL DIS	Hepatitis C negative (8/11); Hep B vaccines completed
ABN KIDNEY FUNCT STUDY	CRI, Neph Dr A; NO NSAIDs**

It sounds like this problem list thing is a lot of work! Yes, it is. As Dr. Doug Meuser says, "It takes so much time, but it makes you *so* much better as a physician." Creating and updating a good problem list is work that is well worth the effort, saving much time down the road and ensuring good patient care and follow-up. I would rather spend the majority of my time cleaning up the problem list than clicking through the chart playing find-and-seek with critical data – and as you will see later, a 99214 only calls for "documenting the status of 3 chronic problems." Your problem list can certainly suffice if your note reflects this effort.

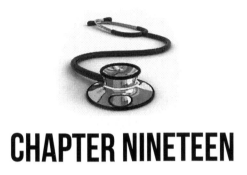

CHAPTER NINETEEN

ROCK STAR SECRETS:

THE EXTREMELY DIRECTED PHYSICAL EXAM

You have obtained your relevant medical history, updating your problem list as you went along. Now on to the Rock Star physical exam.

The Rock Star doctor knows that a "complete" physical examination of an asymptomatic person is a complete waste of time. Yes, I know of the tales of patients being diagnosed early in disease because of an astute clinician picking up a vague physical finding, but what we *don't* hear about are all the sick people who never got seen by a physician at all because their doctor was too full doing complete physical examinations on everyone. Or the patient that had a coincidental finding on examination, which led to painful and unnecessary testing showing that absolutely nothing was wrong.

No one wants to think about personal rationing of health care, but when it comes to populations, the reality is that a complete physical examination is time better spent on evidence-based data collection, history taking, counseling, and preventive care.

This is not to say that good examination skills are not absolutely essential. They are! But the exam needs to be *directed* in a way that maximizes the chance of a correct diagnosis in the minimum of time.

After mastering the complete physical examination in medical school, doctors move on to what we call the "directed" physical examination. This means that instead of examining every body part, we focus on the areas that are relevant to the clinical situation. This is an area that separates students from master clinicians.

A Rock Star physician understands that often the most important element of patient interaction involves listening and discussing a care plan. To perform a detailed examination, especially if there is no clinical relevance, is wasted time that could be spent more effectively. Fortunately, the Rock Star physician becomes a master at the "extremely directed" physical examination, gleaning a wealth of information from careful observation during the office visit. Like a 21st century Sherlock Holmes, the astute physician takes in clinical data at first glance, observing a multitude of examination elements before even laying hands on the patient. Adding in a handshake and watching the patient walk across the examination room adds even more to the clinical picture.

ROCK STAR RULE #7:

Learn to document a physical exam just by looking

Think about it: as you enter the exam room, you immediately take in the patient's state of distress, skin color and texture, conjunctiva, facial symmetry, respiratory effort – all in an instant. In fact, a Rock Star physician can perform an entire focused physical "just by looking."

A JUST-BY-LOOKING PHYSICAL EXAM COULD BE DOCUMENTED:

- Vital signs (taken by your nurse)

- General: acute distress, toxic/nontoxic, well-nourished/hydrated

- Head: normocephalic, atraumatic, symmetric

- ENT: eyelids, eyes/conjunctiva, lips/ mucosa, external ears, hearing

- Neck: range of motion, thyromegaly

- Respiratory: labored or rapid breathing

- Cardiovascular: regular rate (from vital signs), rhythm (if documented by your nurse while taking vitals)

- Abdomen: distended or non-distended

- Extremities: cyanosis, edema

- Skin: obvious rashes, lesions

- Neurologic: cranial nerves, balance, gait, symmetry

A Rock Star physician can document much of the "detailed" examination just by looking at the patient (see Rock Star charting).

Of course, patients don't always realize how much of a physical examination a seasoned physician is doing during what seems to be a casual interaction. A "hands-on" examination – even just a quick auscultation of the heart and lungs – may be necessary to provide that doctoring image that many patients expect, while educating the patient when necessary that a complete physical is no longer considered standard of care.

A patient presenting for depression, for example, needn't be subjected to extensive poking and prodding, which actually cuts into time more worthy of exploring the depression symptoms and treatment options. Or to put it more plainly, a patient with an upper respiratory infection doesn't need a rectal exam.

In fact, current thinking may even go so far as to say that doing unnecessarily detailed examinations may be *harmful* to the patient. How can that be, patients often ask? For every patient "saved" by an amazing physician pick-up, like the palpation of an ovarian tumor, for example, there are many more that go through unnecessary and often invasive testing for irrelevant physical findings. These additional tests can be expensive, painful, and in some cases, lead to adverse consequences like surgical complications. Save the invasive exams for when they are clinically relevant.

It should go without saying that the concept of the extremely directed physical relates to clinical situations that don't require a more detailed examination. The Rock Star physician will always perform a more comprehensive examination when it is indicated.

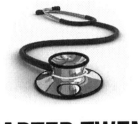

CHAPTER TWENTY

THE GYNECOLOGIC EXAM OR "GET IN, GET OUT"

One of the biggest compliments that I get on my GYN exams is "Wow, that was fast!" In my opinion, a routine pap test shouldn't take longer than 60-90 seconds. Unfortunately, I've personally experienced the prolonged pap test- probably not more than a few minutes, but it seemed like an eternity as I wondered "What is she *doing* in there?"

As with most office procedures, the key to getting a pap done *fast* is to have a standard protocol and to do things the same way, every time. And, of course, practice makes perfect.

If you're an expert with the speculum, you can skip this section. But if your patients aren't complimenting your speedy pap tests regularly, maybe a quick read-through is worthwhile.

1. **Have the room set up**. Your assistant should have the room set up for you with everything that you will need. Your speculum, the smallest size that you need to get the job done, a light source, and your testing material. After the speculum is inserted is *not* the time to be rummaging through drawers for supplies. I keep my assistant in the room with me, but she stands to the side of the exam table for the privacy of the patient.

2. **Make the procedure as comfortable as possible**. Use cloth stirrup covers, drape the patient with linen rather than flimsy paper if possible, and talk in calm, reassuring, but matter-of-fact tones.

3. **"Assume the position."** I like to help guide my patient's heels into the stirrups, extend the stirrups out towards me as far as possible, and then ask the patient to "scootch" down to the very end of the exam table. Keep her draped until the last minute.

4. **Tell the patient what you are doing**. "I'm going to place the speculum now." Having been on the receiving end of an unexpectedly invasive exam during one of my first female exams, I can tell you that lack of fair warning is very disconcerting.

5. **Insert the speculum**. Make sure your patient's bottom is at the extreme end of the exam table. Use very firm inferior pressure (towards the perineum) with the speculum to pass the introitus. Have the patient take deep breaths and not clench her muscles.

6. **Open the speculum only after it is fully inserted**. Again, I let the patient know that the speculum will make a clicking sound when it opens.

7. **With the cervix in view, take your sample** – this should be really quick – hand it off to the nurse, and get the speculum out of there.

8. **Hold forward-pressure on the speculum as you release the handle SLOWLY**, otherwise it will spring back and pinch the patient. Sometimes taking the speculum out is more uncomfortable than putting it in if you aren't careful.

If you followed these steps, you should hear, "That wasn't bad at all."

THE PELVIC EXAM

This is going to be controversial, but I'll go ahead and say it. The annual pelvic exam is not evidence-based.

Yes, I have heard the stories of the ovarian cancer and other serious pathologies that "happened" to be found during a routine pelvic exam. But I've also seen many, many more examples of invasive and unnecessary testing resulting from questionably palpable abnormalities on examinations.

I am *not* referring to symptomatic women. A woman with abnormal vaginal bleeding, pelvic pain or any gynecologic symptom deserves a thorough vaginal and pelvic examination.

But the completely asymptomatic woman does not need to be subjected to unnecessary and potentially painful examinations. In fact, the USPSTF just concurred – pelvics *not* necessary. [47])

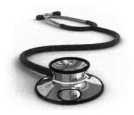

CHAPTER TWENTY-ONE

EXPLAINING THE DIAGNOSIS AND COMMUNICATING THE TREATMENT PLAN

So, you've established the patient and physician agenda for the visit. You've done your directed physical examination. Now it's time to explain the diagnosis and communicate a treatment plan.

The best way that I have found to interact with patients is to stay *positive* whenever possible. Even when discussing a tough diagnosis, putting a positive spin on the information makes it more palatable to the patient and keeps them from shutting down.

For example, telling a patient about a new diagnosis of diabetes: "The good news is that we've caught this early. Now we just need to work together to make the right changes to diet and medication."

It's never a good idea to give difficult news over the telephone. Any new diagnosis warrants a face-to-face visit, allowing time for the patient to digest and to come to terms with this new fact of life.

Keep in mind that patients with medical conditions often feel guilty and ashamed. I try to mitigate some of that shame by emphasizing that while lifestyle is often a major factor, sometimes these disease processes are genetics at work. Such as: "Remember that with your strong family history of diabetes, we have to work harder at weight control."

Focus on the positive changes that your patient has made. If my patient loses one pound, I do a celebratory "Great job!" If they just haven't *gained* any weight, "Good news, you didn't gain any weight during the holiday season." I've been known to give high-fives for an improved BP or A1c. Positive reinforcement works.

Even when we have to get a little "scary" with our patients, we can still keep a positive focus of care and concern. "I'm worried about these elevated sugars. I know that you can do better."

Keeping a team emphasis can really help. Emphasize that you are your patient's ally and that *"we"* are going to work together to get through whatever health issue occurs.

The Rock Star physician keeps in mind that many patients lack health literacy and often have difficulty understanding medical instructions given verbally. It is estimated that with fewer than half of patients remember what the doctor explained by the end of the visit.

To help our patients understand the treatment plan, we may have to focus on a few key points and to repeat these points throughout the visit. This may mean scheduling more frequent follow-up appointments to deal with the various health issues that come up during one visit. Don't forget to be very clear about when you want the patient to follow-up with you. Then schedule that appointment before the patient leaves the office.

Most patients don't understand medical jargon. We have to remember that what is second nature to us as physicians is brand new for most of our patients, especially easily confused terms like "Your test results are negative." To the patient, negative may be taken literally, as in; your test results are bad, while the physician actually means the opposite. It's better to say "Your test results are good, encouraging, etc."

It's really important for our patients to feel comfortable *asking* us to clarify information. I like to say "Sometimes we doctors forget that we are using 'doctor-talk' - stop me at any time if there is anything that I can explain better."

Encourage questions directly – "What questions do you have?" – and have the patient repeat information back to you to confirm understanding. This especially applies to using medical equipment – for example, whenever we teach a patient how to use an asthma inhaler or how to administer insulin, we have the patient practice the technique with the physician or nurse ("see one, do one, teach one!").

Use diagrams, anatomical charts or Internet images to explain the diagnosis better. Showing the sacroiliac area on a musculoskeletal chart is far easier to understand than trying to describe it verbally.

A method that encompasses these strategies is called the "Ask, Tell, Ask" model, and has been shown to help patients digest medical information.[48]

For example, let's take a patient with back pain that you have diagnosed with sacroiliitis.

Doctor: "What do you know about sacroiliitis?" **(ASK)**

Patient: "I've never heard of it."

Doctor: "Sacroiliitis is an inflammation or strain of a joint area in the hip and low back (pointing to a diagram)." **(TELL)**

"Do you see the area I am talking about?" **(ASK)**

Patient: Yes, that's exactly where my pain is.

USE HANDOUTS

Handouts are an extremely important tool for the Rock Star physician. As we discussed previously, most patients fail to remember the majority of what they are told in the exam room. Having a piece of paper with written instructions or helpful advice may make all the difference in the patient's ability to follow the treatment plan.

A clinical summary including names of diagnoses, medication list (and what each medicine is for), and instructions is essential. Even better is to give the patient a copy of the last office note along with the clinical summary incorporating any changes in the plan. If you are able to finish your current office note by the time your patient leaves the office, even better.

Most medical academies and physician websites have medical handouts on a wide array of subjects available to print and give to your patients. I find it useful to create my own handouts on topics that cause the most confusion or that get the most questions. I keep the handouts on my computer, which I can then edit to add additional comments based on patient feedback. For example, if I keep getting a recurring question, I add that information to my handout.

Handouts save the physician time. When referring a patient to physical therapy or psychology, I give a handout with a list of different therapists, including phone numbers and locations, along with instructions on contacting their insurance company to see who is on panel.

ROCK STAR TIP:

Keep forms and hand-outs at your fingertips in the exam room or in an easily accessed holder at the check-out window

I like to jot myself a reminder note at the bottom of the billing ticket ("psychology handout") while I am talking with the patient about the topic so I don't forget. My staff is instructed on what my notes mean so that they can provide the information if I don't.

OFFER TREATMENT OPTIONS

One of the most important ways to communicate the treatment plan is to offer options. I usually say something like: "There are a few things that we can do to help your back pain. We can choose to do nothing and it may get better on its own. We can start you on medication for inflammation. We can also refer you for physical therapy to learn some exercises that may help."

In a study of patient satisfaction, many patients reported liking when their doctors gave them "options," especially alternatives to medication.[49] Offering options gives patients the opportunity to participate in shared decision making, which has been shown to improve patient health outcomes.[50]

Offer reassurance and stay as positive as possible: "You're going to be ok," "We can definitely treat this," "No, you are not going to end up bedridden," or in the case of a more serious diagnosis: "We'll get through this together." As doctors we have a significant influence on patient's perceptions of illness that can last a lifetime.[51] It's very important to set a positive tone for the future.

Encouraging exercise is *always* good – it is surprising how many people are afraid that exercising will make their symptoms worse or will cause them to hurt themselves. Even painless joint clicking/ cracking can cause panic – I like to reassure patients that unless the activity is causing significant discomfort, they simply cannot hurt themselves with exercise.

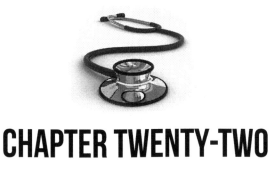

CHAPTER TWENTY-TWO
THE INITIAL PATIENT VISIT

While most of my patient visits are completed in about ten or fifteen minutes, I like to spend a bit longer during an initial patient encounter. This visit is critical to set the tone for the future. It also allows you to develop an accurate chart of the patient's medical history, medication experiences, and problems.

David Voran, MD, says "The goal of a system is to know everything you can about that next *new* patient so you don't have do de-novo data entry." This information will serve as a basis for decision making in the future, and save time down the road.

"You've got to take the time to put in the information at the initial visit – the medical history, not only surgeries but who operated; and then you can carry this information forward at future visits," says Dr. Doug Meuser.

I spend much of my time creating a succinct but detailed problem list (see previous section), which will become the basis for future office visits in patients with chronic medical conditions. I also like to include a history of what medications *haven't* worked and include those on the allergy list – not a true allergy, but as a reminder to me what *not* to prescribe again in the future.

I also like to obtain general information that is easily missed at follow-up visits, like advanced directives, emergency contact information, family relationships, education, employment, etc. These are details that are often included on new patient intake forms and should be entered into your EHR for future reference. I train my staff to input much of this information while they are rooming the patient.

While I generally don't spend long on examinations for my routine patients (other than the directed physical as already discussed), I *do* try to do a more detailed physical on the first visit as a baseline. Generally, a heart murmur isn't going to change without showing some symptoms, so a decent cardiac exam at the first visit will limit the need to auscultate the heart at a routine visit for depression, for example. A "comprehensive" examination is also a requirement for coding a new patient initial visit of 99204 or 99205 (see charting section).

ROCK STAR TIP:

When meeting a new patient, it is essential to obtain medical records from previous physicians and to review these in detail

As internist Beth Shandor, DO, says: "If God is in the details, then old records are God. Records point you in the right direction." Obtaining medical records prevents excessive or unnecessary testing and keeps you from missing important medical details, like past abnormal results.

If your patient has information already in your current electronic medical record (EMR), review the chart in detail. Dr. Jennifer Keehbauch points out: "Once you click on the EMR you are now responsible for everything in it. You've got to get efficient at reviewing the medical chart."

The first visit is an ideal opportunity to explain your office philosophy and protocols. Emily Nabors, MD, has a standard script for meeting new patients, including a brief biography of her training, and followed by an explanation of what a Family Physician is. "I send a handwritten note to every new patient welcoming them to my practice." She includes a magnet with her practice information with the welcome letter.

I use a new patient handout that I created to answer most of the questions that new patients ask.

SAMPLE NEW PATIENT HANDOUT

ROCK STAR MD/DO
ADDRESS, PHONE NUMBER

Office Hours   Monday - Wednesday 7:30 AM to 6 PM
Friday 7:30 AM to 4 PM
Closed on THURSDAYS, weekends and national holidays

Appointments

- Dr. Rock Star will make every effort to maintain your scheduled appointment time, although emergencies may cause a delay. We will do our best to keep you informed of any schedule issues, and will be happy to reschedule your appointment if needed, at your convenience.

- Please arrive 10 minutes prior to your scheduled time to update insurance and other pertinent information.

- Please allow 24 hours when canceling or rescheduling appointments to better accommodate other patients

- Urgent or same-day "sick" visits are always available during routine office hours. If Dr. Rock Star is out of the office, another physician will be covering.

Medications

- Dr. Rock Star will prescribe enough of your routine medications to last until your next scheduled appointment. All new medications require an appointment to discuss risks, benefits, and side effects.

- Appointments are required for all controlled substances (pain medication, sleeping pills, etc.) No refills are permitted without office visit. Controlled substance prescriptions may require signing a medication agreement and random drug tests as required by current state statutes.

Test Results and Telephone Messages

- Dr. Rock Star feels very strongly that all test results including lab and x-ray be explained at a follow-up visit. This is for your benefit and protection, as missing test reports are one of the most frequent cause of medical error in the United States.

- Telephone calls will be returned as soon as possible, no later than 24 hours from the initial call to the office.

Referrals to Other Physicians

- Our office will be glad to schedule an appointment for you with specialty physicians as recommended by Dr. Rock Star. We urge you to keep any scheduled appointments or cancel within a reasonable time frame. We strongly recommend checking with your insurance carrier regarding participating providers.

After Hours Emergency Care

- The local emergency room is open 24 hours per day, and is located at < enter address, phone number.>

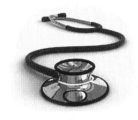

CHAPTER TWENTY-THREE

HEALTH MAINTENANCE

ROCK STAR RULE #8:

Health maintenance: Every visit, every time

In my residency, the mantra "Health maintenance, every visit, every time," was drilled into our heads. Although it is frustrating and challenging to try to crowbar preventive care issues like paps and mammograms into an 8-10 minute visit, the Rock Star doctor must admit that in this case, the profs were right.

Waiting until a "physical" or wellness visit to address health maintenance issues just doesn't work – why? Number one, patients may never actually come in for a wellness visit, only visiting your office for sick visits.

Number two, when they *do* come in for their wellness visit, they often bring up all sorts of chronic and acute issues – and patients don't want to be told "I'm sorry, but we can't discuss your chest pain today; we are only doing your annual wellness visit!"

Thirdly, do you think that the patient (or jury, for that matter) will care that you never recommended that colonoscopy "because the patient never came in for a physical?" All they know is that they've seen you seven times in the last few years for assorted sick visits and no one ever suggested colon cancer screening...

We are expected to do the right thing for our patients, as challenging as that may be. So, the most practical way to overcome these barriers is to wedge preventive care into routine office visits, whenever possible. This means negotiating your medical agenda with your patient's agenda. An efficient problem list can be part of the solution.

And on a positive note, at last we *get paid* for doing health maintenance. Medicare has multiple screening codes to show discussion of depression, alcohol, tobacco, and obesity counseling for example. These codes can be tacked onto routine office visits. In and of themselves, the codes don't pay much. But if you code these services on *all* your appropriate patients, the RVUs start to add up. I will show you in a later section how to create custom questionnaires and tools to efficiently document your screening services and support this additional coding.

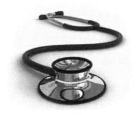

CHAPTER TWENTY-FOUR
THE WELLNESS VISIT AND SCREENING CODES

Now that Medicare and other commercial insurances are paying for an annual preventive or wellness visit (Annual Wellness Visit – AWV), it is in the best interest of the physician and the patient to schedule a visit to review health maintenance.

Medicare covers three versions of the wellness visit. The "Welcome to Medicare" visit (within one year of Medicare eligibility), the initial wellness visit, and subsequent wellness visit.

The Medicare requirements for the wellness exam are listed on the Center for Medicare Services (CMS) website.[52] As guidelines are often changing, be sure to check the website for the most current recommendations. For example, a newer element of the AWV requires patients to fill out a health "patient self-assessment form."

SAMPLE PATIENT SELF-ASSESSMENT FORM: **MEDICARE PREVENTIVE QUESTIONNAIRE**

Since your last visit here:

- Have you been diagnosed with any new medical conditions? ___Yes___No

If Yes, details:_____

- Have you undergone any recent surgical procedures? ___Yes___No

If Yes, details:_____

- Have you had any medication, vitamin, or supplement changes? ___Yes___No

If Yes, details:_____

- Have any close family members developed any serious illnesses? ___Yes___No

If Yes, details:_____

- Have you changed your use / nonuse of tobacco or alcohol? ___Yes___No

If Yes, details:_____

Please describe your current diet (check all that apply):

___ Well-Balanced, Controlled Portions ___Unbalanced ___Excessive Portions

___ Low Salt ___Low Fat ___Low Carbs ___Restricted Calories (_____ cal/ day)

___ Other: _____

Please describe your current activity level:

___ Minimal ___ Active, but No Exercise ___Some Exercise ___Regular Exercise

Have you had an eye examination within the last year? ____Yes ____ No

Name of eye doctor_____

Do you have any difficulties with your hearing? *(Are you unable to hear your fingers rubbing together when you hold your arms outstretched?)*

_____Yes _____Hearing aid   _____ No difficulty

Please list any other doctors regularly involved with your care:

Name _____ Specialty _____

      Phone/Fax if available_____

Name _____ Specialty _____

Phone/Fax if available_____

END OF LIFE CARE

Do you have an Advanced Directive or Living Will? ____Yes ____No

Name/phone # of health care proxy/ surrogate_____

Do you wish to discuss any end-of-life issues during this visit? ____Yes ____No

__Depression Screen :   Do you feel down or depressed? ___ Yes ____No

ACTIVITIES OF DAILY LIVING

Do you need assistance with activities of daily living, such as dressing, grooming, toileting, feeding?

If yes:_____

Do you need assistance with activities such as banking, managing appointments, cooking, shopping?

If yes: _____

SAFETY SCREENING

Do you feel you have any significant safety concerns? ___Yes ___No

Do you have any trouble seeing, hearing, or speaking? ___Yes ___No

Do you have any trouble bathing, dressing, or eating? ___Yes ___No

Do you feel unstable or unsteady when standing? ___Yes ___No

Do you have any trouble using stairs, if you have them? ___Yes ___No

Have you fallen or almost fallen in the last 60 days? ___Yes ___No

Do you know of any hazards in your home? ___Yes ___No

Would you have any trouble getting 911 help if needed? ___Yes ___No

COGNITION SCREENING

Pretend the circle is a clock.

1. Write the numbers on the clock.
2. Mark the time as "11:10"

145

The most efficient way to ensure that you hit all of the required elements of the wellness visit, as required by Medicare, is to create a template to keep you on track. While some electronic medical records may have this at your disposal, many do not. I've created my own patient self-assessment form, based on current guidelines, as well as "macros" for my dictations and documentation of the wellness visit elements.

SAMPLE DICTATION TEMPLATE

WELLNESS VISIT
The patient is here today for an annual Medicare wellness visit.
Current problem list was reviewed in detail. Medications reviewed with patient. Specialists were identified and listed for the patient.
Advanced directives were discussed and records were updated to reflect the patient's wishes.
Cognition was evaluated by the use of a mini cog, and was found to be normal.
Fall risk was reviewed with patient.
Home safety was reviewed with the patient.
Hearing screen- normal, no concerns.
Vision screen-patient is up to date with recent eye exam, and has no new concerns.
ADLs-independent
IADLs-independent
Current diet includes: healthy, low fat diet
Exercise: regular walking
Depression screen: Sadness or depressed mood, anhedonia => denies both
BMI was calculated and reviewed with patient.
A personalized preventive health schedule based on USPS TF recommendations was developed for the patient and discussed in detail. A handout was printed and given to the patient to review.

Dr. Roberta Chung has been using her own forms since before Medicare began covering wellness visits. "I have the patient fill out a self-assessment form once a year. This helps to remind them and me when different screening tests are due."

Patients don't always understand the concept of the wellness exam and the fact that it is not the same thing as a "complete physical." In fact, Medicare currently does *not* require any physical examination, other than review of the body mass index (BMI), blood pressure, and a vision exam for the Welcome to Medicare visit.

To help clarify the intent of the wellness visit, I created a handout to help patients understand the required elements of the visit and to understand that only wellness issues are to be addressed at this time. However, if patients have additional clinical concerns at the time of the wellness visit, there is no restriction on providing that additional care, which should be appropriately billed as a separate E/M visit (with a modifier – 25) along with the wellness code.

In fact, I often do the opposite, tacking on a wellness visit during a routine office appointment for chronic disease management. Since I'm already addressing health maintenance as a matter of routine, all I have to do is have the patient fill out their self-assessment form and print out a preventive health schedule. Voila! I've captured a wellness visit with a minimum of extra effort.

Patients should be aware that while the wellness visit is "free," additional services provided are subject to standard deductibles and copays. Since patients often have chronic medical issues that require attention, or acute problems, they may be addressed at the wellness visit, with an additional bill for these non-wellness elements. I include this information on my wellness visit hand-out. As long as your patients are informed, they should be satisfied, as the alternative is to schedule another appointment on a different day to review any other medical issues.

SAMPLE WELLNESS VISIT INTRODUCTION

Welcome to your annual Medicare Preventive Visit! This exam is intended to help promote your health and identify major risks for disease. Medicare covers this exam once per year. This Medicare benefit has 3 different names based on when it occurs, as follows:

"Initial Preventive Wellness Visit"- also called the "Welcome to Medicare Exam" - available anytime within the first 12 months of joining Medicare

"First Annual Wellness Visit"- available any time after the first 12 months of joining Medicare

"Subsequent Annual Wellness Visit" - available annually after the First Annual Wellness Visit above

Your preventive visit will assess the following:

- your medical and surgical history
- your current medications
- your relevant family history
- your use of any alcohol, tobacco, or illicit drugs
- your current diet and physical activity
- any other physicians involved in your care
- any depression, cognitive impairment, or safety concerns
- an exam of your height, weight, body mass index, BP, & vision, along with any other areas of concern based on the above assessments
- any end-of-life planning concerns

The visit concludes with the following:

- development of a list of any identified preventive health concerns (a problem list)
- education, counseling, and referrals based on any such concerns
- a personalized written screening schedule detailing any recommended screening/preventive services that are covered by Medicare
- recommendations for end-of-life planning, if needed and desired
- other preventive services as may be recommended by your doctor

PLEASE NOTE: Per Medicare, this annual Medicare Preventive Visit is intended to focus on wellness and is limited to health promotion and disease prevention. To the extent that you and your doctor spend any time during your preventive exam addressing non-preventive issues such as illnesses, diseases, and/or injuries that you may have, Medicare has directed us to code and bill for such services separately and in addition to the preventive exam. We mention this in advance of your exam so that you are aware that you may incur charges for this visit, depending on the extent of the exam and any copays and/or deductibles you may be responsible for through your Medicare coverage.

To get started, please complete the following 3 pages of questions, to the best of your ability.

MEDICARE SCREENING AND COUNSELING CODES

Medicare is also now compensating physicians for appropriate screening and counseling. An efficient way to ensure adequate screening is to create a form that all Medicare patients receive once a year (Form 3).

In 2012, Medicare paid $18.25 each time that I screened my patients for depression or alcohol. Not a ton of money, but considering that this screening can be done simply by having the patient fill out a form, doing the screening is a no-brainer. There is also additional reimbursement for counseling patients on smoking cessation, alcohol abuse, obesity, cardiovascular risk reduction, and sexually transmitted diseases. Check the CMS website for the most current guidelines on required elements of counseling and coding rules. If you're doing the work, you might as well get paid for it.

As part of prescreening charts before the patient's visit, your nurse or secretary should check to see when the patient last had a "wellness" visit or screening evaluation. If more than a year has elapsed, the forms should be attached to the patient's ticket for the next day as a reminder to the physician.

One caution: Once I initiated this screening process, I had a rash of patients calling and coming in concerned about being labeled an "alcoholic" or saying "I'm not depressed!" after they received their explanation of benefits (EOB) reflecting payment for screening by Medicare. To explain that the bill simply reflects that I *asked* about depression and alcohol, I added this information at the top of the screening form. While the explanation definitely cut down on patient concerns, I still do get questions from worried patients from time to time. Still well worth doing the screening.

SAMPLE SCREENING FORM

Medicare is requesting that primary care physicians perform annual screenings for depression, alcohol, and cardiovascular disease, as well as provide counseling for patients with identified problems with alcohol, tobacco, or sexually transmitted diseases. Screening for these issues has been shown in scientific studies to benefit health.

In order to demonstrate to Medicare that the screenings are being done, our office transmits a code that Medicare has developed. This code will show up on your "explanation of benefit" form or bill, and will be covered 100% by Medicare with no co-pay or deductible. The code does NOT indicate that you have a problem with alcohol, depression, etc, only that we screened for these issues as required. To comply with Medicare guidelines, Dr. Rock Star would sincerely appreciate if you would fill out this simple form.

Depression Screening		
During the past month, have you often been bothered by:		
1. Little interest or pleasure in doing things?	___Yes	___No
2. Feeling down, depressed, or hopeless?	___Yes	___No
Alcohol Screening (note: 1 drink = 1.5 oz or "shot" of liquor; 5 oz of wine; or 12 oz of beer)		
Do you drink more than 7 drinks per week?	___ Yes	___ No
Do you drink greater than 3 drinks per occasion?	___ Yes	___No
Have you ever felt the need to cut down on drinking?	___ Yes	___No
Does anyone ever annoy you by commenting on your drinking?	___ Yes	___No
Do you feel guilty about drinking?	___ Yes	___No
Do you ever have a morning "eye-opener?"	___ Yes	___ No
Cardiovascular disease screening		
Do you take an aspirin daily?	___Yes	___No
Sexually transmitted disease screening		
Do you have any concerns about STDs?	___Yes	___No
Would you like to have an HIV test?	___Yes	___No
Do you have any of the following risk factors:		
Multiple sex partners, using barrier protection inconsistently, having sex under the influence of alcohol or drugs, having sex for money or drugs, an STD in the last year, IV drug use, or men having sex with men		
	___ Yes	___No

TOBACCO AND ALCOHOL COUNSELING

Medicare also reimburses physicians for counseling on tobacco and alcohol cessation. If you take a few minutes during your office visit to discuss these issues with your patients, be sure to document the discussion and code for the time that you spent counseling.

OBESITY COUNSELING

For patients that have a body mass index (BMI) of 30 or more, physicians can be compensated for counseling on weight reduction. Currently Medicare pays for this code weekly for one month, every two weeks for the next five months, and if your patient has lost at least 3 kg during that time, they will pay for a monthly visit for another six months.

Since the current reimbursement for obesity counseling is about $25 per visit, setting up group visits is a practical way of incorporating weight loss counseling into a busy schedule. I did this for a while in my previous practice, and although I'm not sure that it was a particularly financially beneficial program, my patients loved it, and many of them did lose weight.

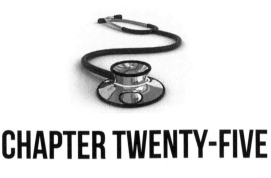

CHAPTER TWENTY-FIVE

GETTING OFF-STAGE

ENDING THE VISIT GRACEFULLY

So, you've engaged with your patient, assessed the medical needs, addressed as many concerns as you can within your limited time frame, reviewed health maintenance, and you're ready to wrap up the visit. *It's time to get out of the exam room.*

As difficult as active listening is, it is often even harder to gracefully *end* listening. Wouldn't it be lovely to have a little buzzer (or in some cases, a trap door!) that could signal that "time's up?" Instead, we have to take the initiative to conclude a visit.

The Rock Star doctor knows how to lead the patient through the office visit, and that includes ending on a positive note. One of the best ways to end a patient visit is to ask, while still seated, and with a tone of sincerity, "Did we miss anything important today?" It is critical to avoid giving the impression of rushing – you know, the old hand-on-the-door routine we docs are well known for.

Although it can be almost painfully difficult to keep your butt in your chair when you are *so* ready to get out of the room and move on to the next patient, you *must* stay seated, leaning forward, and really showing that you care about everything that your patient wants to tell you. Because you are a Rock Star who has given him your complete attention, the patient feels as if you have spent hours with him, and 9 times out of 10 there will be no additional concerns. At least, not important enough that it can't wait until next time.

If your patient continues to list health concerns, it's OK to say something like: "We've covered a lot of territory today – let's set up a follow-up appointment to address any additional issues."

In many cases, the visit will conclude naturally after a discussion of the diagnoses and treatment options. The doctor may write a prescription, order labs or provide educational literature, and either escort the patient to the check-out area to pick up these items or bring in a nurse to conclude the administrative tasks. Either way, the most important way to conclude an office visit is to *get out of the exam room.*

Remember, the longer you sit in the exam room, whether it's writing out orders or completing your note, the more opportunity you give your patient to come up with more concerns, questions or random thoughts. Usually these are items that the nurse or office coordinator can easily answer and should not require physician time such as: "What time does the lab open?" or "Where is the radiology center located?"

One useful technique to get out of room is to bring in an assistant in to wrap things up – your assistant can address any minutia like "Can you change my prescriptions to go to a mail-order pharmacy?" You've trained your assistants to handle prescriptions, samples that were promised, and logistics.

More sinister from a time management perspective are new health complaints that may pop into the patient's mind while she has time to sit quietly as you hammer at the keyboard in the exam room. "While I have you here, doc…" These are items that necessitate another office visit, but they are hard to deflect once the question is out there.

If the patient thinks up these questions with the nurse or at the check-out window, your assistant can set up a follow-up visit to discuss any further issues.

If by some chance you were already on your way out the door and the patient mentions a "by-the-way," drag yourself right back to your chair and sit down, even if just for a second.

ROCK STAR TIP:
Make sure that your patient feels heard, even if you don't take action at today's visit

Ways to communicate that you have heard your patient include statements like: "I'm glad you mentioned that," "I really want to explore that more," and then "Let's schedule a follow-up visit to give 'blank' the time it deserves."

Naturally, we want our patients to express their concerns – just not at the end of the allotted visit time! There are few things worse than that dreaded hand-on-the-doorknob comment, "Oh, I forgot to mention, doctor…" that turns out to be a something that can't be ignored, like chest pain or a recent fainting spell. This after you just spent the last 10 minutes discussing the latest screening test, since the patient initially reported no new health issues!

To prevent these "by-the-way" issues, the Rock Star doctor will try to get the most important health concerns addressed at the beginning of the visit. One way to do this is to have your medical assistant obtain introductory information including the "History of Present Illness." She can type patient complaints into your note, which you can later triage yourself, either adding data, editing details or, in some cases, deleting issues that just can't be addressed on that particular visit.

Asking the patient to bring written lists to their visit can help them to focus and prioritize their concerns, and letting the patient know from the start that you can't address all of his concerns can be helpful. "It looks like we have a lot of territory to cover today. Let's focus on the most important issues, and at the next visit…" This shows that you care about all patient concerns, but won't get to all of them in one visit. It sets expectations and the stage for follow-up planning.

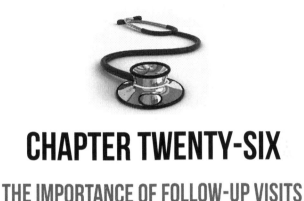

CHAPTER TWENTY-SIX
THE IMPORTANCE OF FOLLOW-UP VISITS

Frequent follow-up is an essential element of chronic disease management. I sometimes have patients in their 70s and 80s who want to come in just once a year ("But I'm perfectly healthy!"), meanwhile they are on 12 different medications! I explain that medications and chronic conditions require ongoing monitoring. Much can change about a person's health in a one-year period and this prevents crisis phone calls in between office visits.

ROCK STAR TIP:

To incentivize patient follow-up, only prescribe enough medication to last until the next scheduled appointment

At the end of the office visit, I request that a follow-up appointment be scheduled at checkout, so that the patient will receive a reminder call. If the Hemoglobin A1c is due in 3 months, medication is prescribed for 3 months. Refills will be given when we review the lab results. After all, the results might cause us to change the prescription!

If the patient needs routine labs on a designated schedule (A1c checks every three months for diabetics, for example), I try to give the lab order for the next blood test as the patient is checking out. However, I only do this if I have the patient in the office, and never by phone. I often have patients calling requesting orders for labs "before my office visit." Not only is ordering labs by telephone uncompensated physician time, but there is too much potential for ordering the wrong tests without having the patient (and her chart) in front of you.

Frequent follow-up also allows the patient time for contemplation of treatment decisions or lifestyle changes. Although your patient may not be ready to quit smoking the first 100 times you told them, they may come in to the next visit and proudly announce that they kicked the habit – "because you told me to, doc!" These rare times are what keep a Rock Star doctor motivated to stay in practice.

Be kind and understanding when your patients present to their follow-up visit without having done *anything* that you advised them to. I used to feel frustrated ("why are they even coming back if they're not going to do anything I said?!") but now I focus on the fact that their presence means that they are still in the "pre-contemplation" phase and, hopefully, at the next visit they will make some progress in improving their health.

Patients often feel guilty themselves when they don't follow their treatment plan. Every day I have a patient that says, "I know you're going to be mad at me, but…". Empathy and understanding will limit guilt as being a barrier to follow-up.

If a patient doesn't seem ready to make changes in their health, you can always include the option of "doing nothing" or contemplation - "why don't you give it some thought/ talk it over with... and we'll discuss it more at the next visit." This keeps the patient from just agreeing with you at the visit and then doing absolutely nothing that you said. We don't want our patients to lie to us just to make us feel better.

When scheduling follow-up appointments, give ranges whenever possible. For example, suggest follow-up in 2-4 weeks; this allows the patient to choose based on their comfort level, as factors affecting follow-up may include money, time off from work, fear/ anxiety, and their schedule.

Never be afraid to see people back sooner, especially if you are concerned about a particular problem. It is not uncommon for me to bring patients back on a daily basis if they have a severe cough or an aggressive wound. A one-week follow-up for a patient with severe life stress can be very appropriate. In my experience, most people are very accepting of scheduling a return visit as they know that their physician is concerned about them.

ROCK STAR TIP:

Always send the patient home with written information

THE WRITTEN SUMMARY

By now we well understand that *patients don't remember half of what they hear at a typical office visit.* Sending the patient home with at least *something* in writing makes a difference.

Ideally, creating a written summary in patient-friendly language will help the patient to understand and remember the medical plan. The medical summary should include the current medication list and future plan. I also like to include the problem list, any instructions I gave the patient, the follow-up dates, and the tests that I have ordered. I encourage the patient to take this summary to all other doctor appointments to share information.

If you can't get your electronic record to print a meaningful summary, send the patient home with a print out of their last office visit or even just jot a few notes on a prescription pad or a blank piece of paper. Anything written is better than nothing.

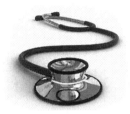

CHAPTER TWENTY-SEVEN

OFFICE FLOW AND MAXIMIZING PATIENT-PHYSICIAN FACE-TO-FACE TIME

ROCK STAR RULE #9:

Maximize patient-physician face-to-face time

While we all complain about the administrative hassles of medicine, most physicians agree that the best part of their medical practice is time spent with patients. Since patient care is what we like (and what we're good at!), the Rock Star physician will set up a practice that maximizes patient interaction and minimizes anything that is not direct patient care.

One way to achieve office efficiency is to use a "lean" system that focuses on minimalist workflow. The lean system is borrowed from manufacturing protocols like the Toyota Production System and involves a concept called "value-stream mapping."[53]

This is essentially a fancy term for drawing a map of office flow in an attempt to identify and remove wasteful steps in the process.[54] And there certainly are unnecessary tasks. Check this out: In an office analysis of primary care work flow, 191 separate tasks were identified in standard office care, including 12 "major" tasks and 189 "subtasks."[55] Somewhere along those 191 tasks, there must be room for streamlining!

If you're like most doctors, you can already identify a half dozen unnecessary steps or "time-sucks" in your office flow. The challenge is finding *where* you can implement change. For example, it may not be feasible to knock down existing walls to locate exam rooms closer together. Or you may be obligated to utilize an electronic system with multiple log-in procedures, wasting valuable minutes with each patient encounter.

And of course, transforming any element of your practice requires significant "buy-in" from the medical team. For employed physicians, rarely empowered to make change, suggestions for process transformation may be stalled due to red tape and office bureaucracy. However, you may be able to identify unnecessary tasks through a workflow analysis that can be resolved with a simple fix.

ROCK STAR FIXES TO MAXIMIZE PHYSICIAN-PATIENT FACE-TO-FACE TIME

EXAM ROOMS

So, let's focus on some simple ways to maximize physician-patient face-to-face time. First, a busy primary care physician needs at least 3, and preferably 4, exam rooms. As you leave one exam room, you should be able to walk right into the next exam room without having to wait for your assistant to do data entry, take vitals, etc. Organize exam rooms to save steps – they should be clustered together and close to the reception area.[56]

Each exam room should be fully stocked with standard supplies, as well as commonly used patient education materials. The doctor should not have to leave the exam room to find what she needs. Labels are helpful to identify the location of supplies. Also, each exam room should have the same layout if possible.

Good communication, especially nonverbal cues, is essential to maintain flow with multiple clinical staff members. A flag system should be posted at each exam room to identify where the physician and medical staff are at any given time. Each flag identifies the person in that particular exam room – we have a "patient," "nurse," and "physician" flag. We also have an "orders" flag to identify patients waiting for a nurse to give an injection, draw blood, etc. When all of the exam rooms are full, we also use a special marker to identify the "next" room ready for the physician. This minimizes the need for verbal communication.

A "white board" can be stationed in the nurse area cueing the staff as to where to go next. I jot notes like, "B12 #2" or "Labs #3" on the board so that I can move on to the next room without having to wait for a nurse to appear.

I also like to write notes on the bottom of the billing ticket for any tasks I need my clerical assistant to help with: "Referral Dr. Smith Neurology for worsening headaches" or "Give samples of Medicine X." I also note a time frame for follow-up so that an appointment can be scheduled at check-out.

MANAGING PHONE CALLS

Telephone calls are a major source of interruption in workflow. It is critical that the Rock Star physician keep phone calls to a minimum. You don't want to spend the time that you could be seeing patients in the office on the phone, nor do you want your nurse tied up answering clinical questions. Instead, patients should be well educated at the office visit and asked to schedule a return visit for any concerns, questions or changes in their symptoms. At the time of this writing, there is no reimbursement for telephone calls, and for other than the quickest question patients should be coming in to see the physician for any concerns.

The Rock Star physician will empower his staff to handle most telephone calls. Each physician should create a triage protocol and encourage a low threshold for making appointments.

Staff should never interrupt the physician in the exam room for a phone call. One exception is phone calls from another physician or medical office. My staff knows to come and get me out of a room for these calls – otherwise the ensuing phone tag will create an even worse time drag.

Restricting phone calls isn't about being a "greedy" doctor: it's about practicing good medicine. Medical standards demand that patient care involve an examination (even if it's just looking) and adequate record keeping. Both of these are limited by telephone encounters. Until technology creates an ideal telemedicine system with video conferencing (and recent studies on this model aren't very encouraging as far as clinical success and patient satisfaction), the face-to-face office encounter is mandatory in providing medical recommendations and treatment.

Following medical standards is critical to maintain your medical license – and, therefore, your livelihood. When questioned by my patients who can't understand why I can't just "call in" a prescription, I am never hesitant to remind them that both their health and my medical license are on the line.

PHONE CALLS WHEN "ON CALL"

As discussed above, telephone consultations are not appropriate for diagnosing and treating medical conditions. Being "on-call" provides an opportunity to educate patients that after-hours phone calls are generally going to result in one of the following answers: 1. Go to the Emergency Room. 2. Call the office on Monday.

No, I won't refill your Percocet. No, I won't call in antibiotics for your cold. If you're worried enough to call the doctor, you need to be seen and examined by a physician.

Consistency in handling after-hours calls is essential for everyone in the physician group, as "giving in" to medication refills, etc. will only encourage more calls like this in the future. Create an office policy as a group and *stick to it!*

DEALING WITH MEDICATION REFILLS

Phone calls for medication refills take up a *ton* of unreimbursed staff time in the typical physician office. It is helpful to try to prescribe enough medication to last until the scheduled follow-up visit. If the patient runs out early, schedule a follow up visit and only prescribe enough to last until that visit. This will discourage repeated phone calls for medication refills outside of office visits.

Now no one is advocating withholding essential medications until an office visit. Except in the case of controlled substances, it is not unreasonable to call in a short-term supply of routine medications until the patient can come in for a visit. For example, you wouldn't let a young woman run out of her birth control because she is a few months overdue for her pap test or a diabetic patient run low on insulin because the Hemoglobin A1c isn't back yet.

However, withholding refills is a practical way of ensuring follow-up visits during the appropriate time interval. As Carlos Portu, MD, says, "If the A1c is due in 3 months, I expect the patient back in that time frame."

It is our responsibility as a physician to ensure adequate follow-up. Continuously refilling medications without an office visit is dangerous and a potential source of liability.

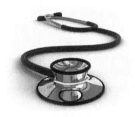

CHAPTER TWENTY-EIGHT
CONTROLLED SUBSTANCE PRESCRIBING

Speaking of medical refills, one of the most common phone calls I get is for a refill on controlled substances, despite the fact that I have a clear policy that these meds won't be refilled without an office visit. It is essential to have established office policies for prescribing controlled substances and to strictly stand by your policy. I have included this information on my new patient welcome form.

Prescribing controlled substances is a particular challenge for most physicians. Some physicians have become so frustrated by "seeking" patients or terrorized by legal threats that they have declined to prescribe any controlled medications at all.

But what then happens to the patient with a broken ankle who has to wait to see the orthopedist? Or the patient with end-stage COPD that could receive relief with a small amount of morphine? Judicious prescribing of controlled medications is one of our responsibilities. Therefore we need to develop our own policies and standards to help us balance this with the risks of prescribing.

It can be very helpful to use resources like the *"SCOPE of Medicine – Safe and Competent Opioid Prescribing Education"* program[57]. This website includes sample pain contracts, tools to evaluate opioid misuse, and patient safety information.

All patients receiving chronic controlled medications should receive drug-specific informed consent, sign and abide by a controlled substance contract, and be monitored as appropriate by random pill counts, urine toxicology testing, and state database review.

Drug tests are a very important tool – not only can they show inappropriate medication use, but can also help determine if the patient is actually taking her medication as prescribed. For example, a negative urine drug test in a person reporting regular use of controlled substances should raise a red flag for diversion of that medication.

Any inappropriate use of controlled medications should result in no further prescriptions for controlled substances. And flagrant abuse of your trust as a physician should result in dismissal from the practice.

DRUG ENFORCEMENT AGENCY (DEA) CONTROLLED SUBSTANCE SCHEDULES[58]

You may already know everything there is to know about controlled substances, but for recent graduates/ new doctors, there may be questions on when narcotics can be faxed, which ones can be refilled, etc. Here are the basics of prescribing controlled substances from the DEA.

Controlled substances are classified into five categories or schedules based on medical indication and abuse potential. Schedule I drugs are the most dangerous class of drugs and are generally illegal and not available for general prescribing. Unless you're in a marijuana-legal state, forget about Schedule I's.

Schedule II drugs have a high potential for abuse, potentially leading to severe psychological or physical dependence. Examples of Schedule II drugs are Attention Deficit Disorder (ADHD) drugs like methamphetamine, and pain medications like morphine, methadone, hydromorphone (Dilaudid), oxycodone (Percocet, OxyContin), and fentanyl (Duragesic). Hydrocodone was recently changed from a category III to a category II drug.

Schedule II drugs cannot be refilled and can never be called in. However, the physician may issue multiple prescriptions for a total of a 90-day supply of a schedule II controlled substance if appropriate. The prescriptions must provide written instructions on each indicating the earliest date on which a pharmacy may fill them ("fill date").

Prescriptions for Schedule II medications may be faxed ahead to the pharmacy, but the original (or "hard copy") prescription must be presented to the pharmacist by the patient prior to the actual dispensing of the controlled substance. Exceptions to the "hard copy" requirement include residents of Long Term Care Facilities and Hospice patients.

Schedule III drugs have a moderate potential for physical and psychological dependence. Commonly used Schedule III drugs are codeine and testosterone. These medications may be faxed, but not called in to a pharmacy. They may be refilled up to five times in six months.

Schedule IV drugs are thought to have a lower potential for abuse and dependence (although many physicians find this debatable), such as hypnotics like zolpidem (Ambien) and benzodiazepines like alprazolam (Xanax). Tramadol (Ultram) was recently changed from a schedule V to a schedule IV. These medications may be called in or faxed, and may be refilled up to five times in six months.

Schedule V drugs have a low potential for abuse and include preparations containing limited quantities of certain narcotics like cough syrups or antidiarrheals, as well as pain medication pregabalin (Lyrica). These medications may be called in or faxed and they may be refilled up to five times in six months.

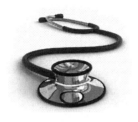

CHAPTER TWENTY-NINE

DEALING WITH LAB RESULTS — "NO NEWS IS NOT GOOD NEWS!"

A frequent phone call that physician offices receive is for lab results. In my opinion, the very best policy for lab tests is a face-to-face visit to review the results in detail. There are many reasons why this policy is ideal for both the patient *and* the physician.

1. **An office visit ensures that the physician has received *all* test results.** It is frighteningly common to find that lab results have been filed before being seen by the physician, that specimens were lost by the laboratory or that they simply disappear into cyber-space (what I call "computer limbo"). Missing lab and radiology reports are a major cause of malpractice suits in the United States. The *only* way to ensure that patient results are

received in their entirety is to review the results in person with the patient. I don't care how many tickler files, computer in-box tasks or other reminder systems you have in place. Eventually, something gets lost or misplaced. And you just have to hope and pray it's not something serious.

2. **An office visit allows you the time to explain results to the patient in detail.** Patient portals, which are computer sites that allow patients to view test results, are now becoming commonplace. The government has even cleared the way to mandate that labs and offices provide patients with lab results. I fully agree that patients need to have access to their results. However, the results should be reviewed with the ordering physician. Inevitably, there will be some minor abnormality – like an elevated MCV or BUN – that may cause the patient concern, triggering a phone call. An office visit will alleviate any concerns about results.

3. **Answer questions about the results.** "What does BUN mean? What should my LDL be?" There will almost always be questions about test results. An office visit is the perfect place to address any questions or concerns.

4. **Follow-up on the clinical issues that prompted the lab orders in the first place!** Example: A 24-year-old woman comes into your office for "fatigue." After obtaining the history and doing a physical, you don't have an explanation for the fatigue, so you order lab results – a CBC, CMP, TSH – which all return normal. The patient calls for results. Saying "everything is OK," doesn't explain *why* the patient has fatigue. The return visit is not just a time to review lab results, but an opportunity to further explore the differential diagnosis of the underlying complaint. Often, once physiologic problems have been ruled out, the patient may now be ready to consider alternate causes of her fatigue and may

share additional information with you, such as psychological stressors.

5. Act on any abnormal results. 'Nuff said.

TRACKING TEST RESULTS

Tracking test results is a major challenge, consuming a significant amount of physician time. Missing or failure to follow up on results is a leading cause of malpractice claims. According to one study, 7% of abnormal lab results were not acted on and using an electronic health record only *worsened* poor systems.[59]

"It's a logistical administrative nightmare," says Dr. Roberta Chung, who keeps all lab results in a folder until the patient returns for follow-up. Other doctors use computerized tools – Dr. Jennifer Keehbauch has the advantage of a patient portal that allows her patients to log in to review their results. However, she says "I always close the loop on abnormalities and diagnostic tests." For tests that are due in the future, like 6-month mammograms or repeat pap tests, Dr. Ariel Cole says "I send myself a postdated email to make sure that I follow up in the appropriate interval."

The medical literature suggests various techniques, like tickler files, using electronic systems, and allowing patients to obtain their own results without visiting the ordering physician. However, each of these ideas has its own hazard – tickler files require constant monitoring and are prone to human error, electronic systems often lack the ability to interface and need to be programmed properly, and having patients review their own is fraught with danger as they won't have the ability to interpret them properly or be aware of any necessary follow-up.

A study in the Journal of Family Practice showed that a single entry system is inadequate to track results. The study recommended a dual method, using both a log book and lab slip orders. The cost analysis for this recommended system showed a cost of $5.19 per set of tests ordered for each individual patient! The study also concluded "we were unsuccessful in identifying a method that is effective for the follow-up of abnormal laboratory test results. Our guess is that this will require some kind of tickler file system with postcards sent to patients who appear to have not followed up as suggested."[60] Really??

So what is a busy Rock Star physician to do?

For some scenarios, a tickler system is manageable. Pap test results or skin biopsies are not so burdensome that they can't be tracked. I also use this system for follow-up mammograms or other imaging tests that call for a repeat at a certain interval. Lab results, on the other hand, tend to be numerous and complex. Even if the physician thinks she has seen and reviewed the results, what if there is a missing test amongst the ordered labs? It is too easy to miss a result and there are too many questions that may come up.

For me, the decision is clear. Patients *must have* a follow-up visit to discuss lab results. Patients don't always like this, or understand the rationale. It's our job to explain the importance of follow-up. That means coming in to review test results in detail with the ordering physician.

"Absolutely no results over the phone," says Dr. Emily Nabors. "I always ask patients to come back in for lab results," agrees Roberta Chung, MD. "It's just good medicine."

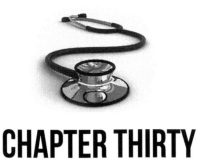

CHAPTER THIRTY

PRIOR AUTHORIZATIONS AND OTHER FORMS

Unreimbursed administrative work is one of the most frustrating elements of clinical practice. Doctors are constantly bombarded by medication refill requests, care coordination letters from insurance companies, and one of the most draining and time-killing tasks: prior authorizations.

Prior authorizations (PAs) are a major burden for primary care physicians. The Journal of the American Board of Family Medicine found that the cost per physician for PA's ranged from $2,161-$3,430 per year[61]. In 2006, PCPs spent 1.1 hours per week on authorizations, nursing staff spent 13.1 hours, and clerical staff 5.6 hours. [62]

A prior authorization, if you haven't had the pleasure, is a form that justifies why the physician feels that a patient needs a particular medication. In the past, prior auths were occasional – a particularly expensive drug or an off-label use of a medication. As insurance companies become more aggressive with cost-saving practices, prior authorizations have almost become the "new norm."

Sometimes prior authorizations are perfectly reasonable – as the prescribing physician, you have decided that a patient needs a non-preferred medication for a particular indication. In this case, the request is easily justifiable, you document a brief explanation, and the medication is usually authorized. Annoying, but not the end of the world. The problem occurs when every other prescription you write bounces back with a prior authorization request, even for generic, inexpensive medications!

THE MAJOR CHALLENGES:

Problem: Prior authorization is requested for a medication started by a previous physician. A new patient comes to you with a long list of medications, requesting refills. He has done well on these medications for some years. You send off the prescriptions. And later that day you get a notification from the pharmacy that the insurance company is declining coverage, demanding an explanation of "why" the patient needs these particular meds.

Now the onus is on the current physician to try to determine what previous medications have been tried, why other medications aren't appropriate, etc.

Solution: Recall the patient. "I'm sorry that I have to bring you back to the office so soon, but I need additional information from you so that I can get your medications authorized by the insurance." Your patient is in the best position to explain his medication history. Thus, filling out the prior auth form with the patient's help is the best way of either getting coverage or finding a different, insurance-preferred medication.

Problem: The medication is on the "Beers" list of medications to be avoided in the elderly.[63] This is a biggie in recent years. Some insurance companies are denying every single medication on the Beers list, which is quite extensive--even when the medication is extremely inexpensive.

Think about every 65-year-old patient that has a once a year prescription for a few Ambien, Xanax, Flexeril, or meclizine.

The insurance company gets to look like they are looking out for the patient's best interest and they save big money when factoring in the sheer volume of these prescriptions.

I have found that PA's just don't work in these cases. While I discourage the use of most drugs on the Beers list, there are some patients for whom they may be the best option for improving quality of life. In this case, I suggest paying out-of-pocket, especially since many of these drugs are quite affordable using a "big box" discount pharmacy.

Solution: Recall the patient and discuss options, including the choice of "paying out of pocket."

FILLING OUT FORMS

Work related to patients not physically present in the office accounted for one fifth (23%) of the average physician's workday, according to the *Annals of Family Medicine.*[64] Of course, none of this time spent working is compensated time.

Much of this work involves filling out forms. The sheer volume of forms that the primary care physician receives each day is astounding. And these forms are rarely less than one page long.

COMMON FORMS

- Prior authorizations for medications, radiology tests

- Disabled parking permits

- Work/ school excuses or return to work permission

- Jury duty excuses

- Family Medical Leave Act (FMLA)

- Nursing home certifications

- Home health certifications

- Physical therapy "plan of care" forms

- Disability insurance or Social Security Disability

- Life insurance forms

- Immigration forms

- Workman's compensation

- Camp forms

- Sports team participation forms

- Department of Transportation (DOT) certifications

- Employment "physical" forms

- Referrals

- Patient assistance program paperwork

The best strategy for dealing with this mountain of paperwork is to require an office visit to fill out forms. This technique allows reimbursement for time spent. And it also helps the physician fill out the paperwork with the best accuracy.

Charles W. Neal, MD, Family Physician from Mount Vernon, IL follows this strategy. "The patient needs to be present for all forms to be filled out. I personally fill out all forms and it is a rare day that I touch any form without the patient present in the exam room with me. Often times I find the patient can help me answer the questions and they appreciate being a part of the process and can better understand the frustrations with me."

Another option is to delegate the work of forms to nursing or clerical staff. This may work for papers that require minimal information, such as dates of service, but becomes more difficult when medical opinion is needed. Often I have my staff fill out as much as possible and then bring the patient in to finish answering medically-related information. While some offices are charging patients for paperwork on a case-by-case basis,[65] I find that this is not usually well-received by patients and certainly is not reimbursable by insurance. The best solution: Bring 'em in.

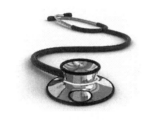

CHAPTER THIRTY-ONE

CLINICAL CHALLENGES IN MEDICINE – ROCK STAR SOLUTIONS

We've dealt with Rock Star solutions to many of the administrative challenges in medicine – now let's move on to clinical issues. One of the biggest frustrations that physicians experience outside of administrative issues is coping with the day-to-day drain of clinical conundrums. From emotionally challenging patients to the daily grind of navigating the health care system, sometimes our work day can feel like "death from a thousand paper cuts," as my Physician Assistant Peter Lindland used to say.

One of the most common daily challenges for physicians is dealing with patients who choose not to follow your carefully considered medical advice.

THE "NONCOMPLIANT" PATIENT

The term noncompliant is out of vogue, as it has an inflammatory connotation. While noncompliance is a good descriptive word for a patient that doesn't do what you want him to, it doesn't adequately sum up the multitude of reasons why this might be the case. It also presumes that you, as the physician, are right about what you want the patient to do, which may or may not be true.

There are many reasons why a patient may be termed as noncompliant. Sometimes they *want* to do the "right" thing, but are simply unable to do so, because of barriers like finances or resources. Maybe they don't really understand what you want them to do or are afraid of the consequences. Therefore, they don't comply. It's possible that you haven't built up enough trust for a therapeutic relationship yet. It is less common for a patient to choose not to comply with your recommendations just because they want to be belligerent. If this were the case, why do they keep coming back to see you?

When you find yourself labeling a patient as noncompliant, ask yourself critically why this might be the case and what your responsibility is both in creating and solving the problem.

WHEN THE PATIENT DOESN'T TAKE YOUR ADVICE

Don't be upset if the patient doesn't take your advice on the first visit. Often the physician has to play salesperson and build a case for a particular treatment plan. It's ok to give the patient some time to process – and ultimately it is his or her decision.

"Patients have to believe in the treatment that you are prescribing," says Jennifer Keehbauch, MD. "You have to convince them why they need to take this medication. Older people will sometimes follow your advice just because you told them to, but the younger generation is 'show me' – they want proof that this is going to work."

When patients decline your recommendations, offer advice in a gentle way - "There are lots of things that we can do to try to help this problem, just so you know... let me know if you ever want to try anything." This sets the stage or plants the seed for possible future interventions.

I also like to say, "It's my job to give you the options and explain the risks and benefits, and it's your job to decide how you want to proceed." As long as the patient at least lets me give them my spiel on a particular medical topic I am satisfied, at least until the following visit.

And if your patient still seems reluctant to pursue your recommendations, avoid expressing anger or frustration. Sometimes after the umpteenth appointment your patient will suddenly agree to your recommendations. "I finally decided to get that colonoscopy, doc." It could be that a friend was diagnosed with colon cancer or it may just be that the patient is finally ready to follow your advice.

In fact, according to a study in the Permanente Journal, patients liked it when a physician "urged them gently to agree to important tests, medications, or procedures even though the patient was [initially] reticent." [66]

Accept that patients aren't always seeing you for your advice, recommendations, treatment, etc. - but rather they want to talk, vent, say what's on their mind or be validated. Sometimes just listening and then saying: "Is there anything I can do to help?" is enough.

And when your patient doesn't take your advice, do what Roberta Chung, MD, advises: "Document, document, document."

OBEY "THE GOLDEN (OR PLATINUM) RULE"

Obviously the Golden Rule: "Do unto others as you would want done unto you" is a well-known and respected adage for good reason. How can you go wrong medically if you are doing what you would do for yourself?

Well, what if you and the patient have different ideas of what you want done?

Paul Marsolek endorses what he calls the "Platinum Rule: Do unto others the way *they* want to be done." In other words, find out what the patient wants done for them. Then use this as your guiding force.

"When my wife is sick," says Mr. Marsolek, "she wants to be pampered, checked in on, brought soup, 'poor-babied.' When I'm sick, I just want to be left alone! If I did to her what I want done for me, she wouldn't be happy, and vice-versa."

Finding out ahead of time and asking permission is the best way to establish a plan of action for medical care. You might be surprised by what you hear. And it will save confusion when the patient doesn't follow a treatment plan that you thought would be best, based on your own preferences.

KEEP COST IN MIND

Sometimes patients don't follow treatment advice because they are concerned about the cost. One third of Americans have trouble paying for medications[67], and 18% of chronically ill patients underuse medications due to cost.[68]

Unfortunately, many patients are reluctant to tell their physician that they are concerned about cost. In a survey of older patients with chronic illnesses, two-thirds did not tell their doctor that they couldn't afford a medication. Instead, they cut back on the dosing to save money.[69] The majority of these patients reported that they didn't discuss costs because they weren't asked about their ability to pay for their medications, and *didn't think that their doctor would be able to help them anyway.*

How sad, when there are so many creative ways of saving on health care costs. Here's how to help:

1. **Ask your patients if they are having any trouble paying for their medications.**

2. **Use generics or lower cost medications whenever possible.** If a branded drug is necessary, look for copay cards on the drug website (for commercial patients – these don't work for Medicare or Medicaid) and consider providing samples. Since many medications are flat-priced, pill splitting can cut costs in half. Consider helping your patients with pharmaceutical assistance programs, usually available on the manufacturer's website. I print the forms off of the Internet and ask the patient to return them filled out and with any required financial information. We then fax the forms and prescription to the pharmaceutical company.

3. **Check prices.** I use a website called www.goodrx.com to check drug prices, especially when I anticipate that insurance will not cover a product or if the patient has no coverage or a high deductible plan. It is often shocking how drug prices change over time (strangely, I have seen several generics *go up* in price) and vary from pharmacy to pharmacy. Sometimes price can be affected by something as minor as the dose. Generic fenofibrate, for example, costs twice as much in the lower 145 mg dose than in the 160 mg dose. Weird.

4. **Use "big box" pharmacies.** In general, warehouse pharmacies like Costco and Sam's Club offer the lowest prices. And, where required by state law, club membership is not needed to use the pharmacies. Low prices can also be found at large stores like Wal-Mart, Target, and some grocery stores. In my experience, self-contained pharmacies like Walgreens and CVS pharmacies tend to have higher prices, although conveniences like 24-hour accessibility may be worth the extra cost at times.

5. **Give 90-day prescription supplies for mail-order pharmacies, when available**. Usually patients get a discount for using these programs.

ANCILLARY TESTING – CONSIDERING COST

Another costly aspect of medical care is ancillary testing. In medical school and residency, little attention is paid to the cost of the tests that we order. Our focus is on learning how to diagnose illness, not on the bottom line. Once we enter into the real world outside of academic medicine, sticker shock becomes a major factor. The costs of laboratory and radiology tests can put a significant financial strain on patients and thus may be a barrier to patient compliance.

"Ordering tests without regard to priority is one of the biggest deficiencies in the junior learner," says Dr. Meuser, UCF and FSU faculty member. "A well-thought out differential diagnosis is essential – 'Ask yourself what concern am I answering by seeking this data, whether it's historical, physical examination, or testing.'"

Make sure that you have an adequate diagnostic code for the tests that you are ordering to avoid denials from insurance companies. Although often requested by patients, there is no such thing as "routine labs." Unless specifically recommended, such as screening lipid panels, most lab tests are not covered without a diagnostic indication.

Of course, lab monitoring is indicated in following many medical conditions, and certain symptoms may warrant laboratory tests. "Fatigue," if present, for example, will usually buy you the whole shebang – CBC, CMP, TSH, B12. Watch out for pricey tests like Vitamin D levels – they aren't covered unless matched by a covering code. "Myalgia and myositis," a common complaint, is acceptable, as are certain other medical conditions. Check your Medicare Local Coverage Determination Policy for the current guidelines.

As with medications, lab prices can vary widely depending on the facility. A little research in my area found that a small local laboratory provided in-house testing at a fraction of the cost of larger labs in the area, with a transparent price list so that patients know ahead of time what the financial obligation will be.

Many radiology sites will also provide discounts for cash or self-pay patients that can be quite remarkable. An MRI that might bill out at over a thousand dollars may only be a few hundred if paid at time of service, for example. A few phone calls to local facilities will help you get a gauge on what the tests you order will cost your patients. Also watch for special pricing, like discount mammograms during October, Breast Cancer Awareness month.

Avoid ordering unnecessary tests, even when requested by your patient. I often have patients requesting "a full body scan" or "complete labs." Again, it is our responsibility to explain why certain tests are not medically necessary, and can actually cause more harm than good in the form of false positives. With the recent media exposure of the Prostate Specific Antigen (PSA) tests, I am finding that patients are starting to understand the concept and danger of false positive tests, which makes education easier.

COMPLIANCE - MAKE IT EASY

One of the best ways to promote compliance with the medical plan is to provide as much one-stop shopping as possible. Offering phlebotomy services in your office is a very welcomed service for most patients and ensures that your patient actually gets the labs done that you've ordered. If labs are needed, do them at the same visit if possible.

Provide directions/maps to local radiology centers and labs if done off-site. Include hours of operation and telephone numbers. Write any necessary instructions clearly on orders – *"Do not eat after midnight"* or *"Must have full bladder for ultrasound,"* for example.

The same goes for referrals: Help your patients schedule with specialists – provide information about the specialist's office: address, phone number, and directions.

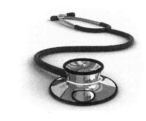

CHAPTER THIRTY-TWO

CLINICAL ISSUES - DEALING WITH CHALLENGING PATIENTS

While it can be fatiguing to help the average patient comply with medical recommendations, dealing with the particularly challenging patient can be even more difficult. I find that in medicine, some days seem to have their themes. One day might be "diabetes day" or "flu day." Every now and then, I seem to have "challenging patient day." You know those kinds of days – when you look at the schedule and groan.

On a typical day, most of us experience one or two difficult patients. A few personality issues can really affect your day and it is much more stressful and mentally draining to have a full day of one challenging patient after the other.

Approximately 15% of patient encounters in adult primary care are considered "unusually difficult" from the physician's perspective.[70] Difficult patients tend to have higher rates of psychiatric conditions and abrasive personality traits. They also are more likely to report multiple physical symptoms with no clear medical explanation. They have higher health care utilization and are more frequently dissatisfied with their medical care.[71] Is it any wonder why these patients induce physician stress?

Some doctors are more stressed by these types of patients -- those who work in larger medical groups, work longer hours, and have less control over the administrative aspects of their practice tend to be more frustrated. Younger physicians, possibly because of less clinical experience, are more easily frustrated, as are those with above average levels of stress, anxiety, and depression. Physicians with more substance-abusing patients tend to be particularly frustrated.

Interestingly, more complex medical problems are *not* associated with increased frustration. Instead, doctors who have more patients with multiple *nonspecific* medical complaints or somatization tend to have increased levels of stress and present a particular mental health challenge to physicians.[72]

Fortunately, there are Rock Star secrets to managing these types of patients while reducing our own stress levels.

CHARACTERISTICS OF THE CHALLENGING PATIENT

- Personality issues, ranging from mild anxiety disorder to the extreme of borderline personality

- Patients that don't follow the treatment plan (noncompliant)

- Poor communicators – either talking excessively on tangents or those who make you drag every detail out of them

- Extremely ill patients with multiple comorbidities

- Diagnostic dilemmas or vague complaints – "dizziness" and "syncope" come immediately to mind

What doctors find challenging can vary from physician to physician. Some doctors enjoy managing day-to-day problems and find diagnostic mysteries stressful, while others like Doug Meuser, MD, find a day of routine coughs and colds extremely boring and mentally unchallenging. "I can't spend all day seeing kids with colds and bronchitis, explaining why antibiotics aren't indicated for viral infections. That's like Hamburger Hill to me – I'll just die on it." Meanwhile, he thrives on musculoskeletal problems, an area that many primary care docs would rather turf out to orthopedics.

When it comes to dealing with challenging patients, we also have to remember that being only human ourselves, we bring our own personality issues and life experiences to the table – as a person who copes with anxiety (or as I like to call it, "extreme Type A personality disorder"), an anxious patient can trigger those feelings in me.

A physician who has had personal experiences with depression, alcohol or drug issues, abuse or family stresses may find dealing with these patient situations to be extremely challenging. Sometimes the way we cope with our own emotions will manifest in our patient interactions – occasionally in obvious ways, but more often in more subtle manifestations. Feelings of inadequacy can evoke emotions like irritability or even anger in coping with an extremely ill patient because of our own sense of anxiety or fear of making a mistake.

The Rock Star doctor must develop a game plan to cope with and learn to help even the most challenging patient.

"WINNING" THE PATIENT OVER

Developing a therapeutic physician-patient relationship is critical in all medical practice, but particularly so in primary care. Unlike work in an urgent care or emergency department, we have the privilege of getting to know our patients over an extended time period and that relationship doesn't necessarily happen right away.

Many challenging patients have had negative experiences with the health care system in the past, either personally or through a friend or family member. We need to remember that we not only have to develop our own relationship, but also that we have to overcome any stigma that was created by former relationships.

ROCK STAR TIP:
The Rock Star physician finds a way of winning the patient over by the basics: *listening, patience, and frequent follow-up visits.*

LISTENING

Listening is addressed in great detail in an earlier section of this book. Ultimately, listening is one of the most important tools for any patient encounter, but in particular for the challenging patient.

Often, previous physicians may have struggled with this individual as well and the patient may feel that he or she has never been properly listened to. This is something that I hear day in and day out, "You're the first person who has ever listened to me." Just allowing the time for this person to express himself in a way that has never been possible before may enable a previously challenging patient to become a pleasant encounter.

PATIENCE

As a physician, it can be so hard to have patience, especially when your mind is filled with other tasks or issues yet to be done. This is especially true when dealing with a challenging patient who may have trouble getting to the point or one who is resistant to recommendations.

The key to developing patience is to use the opportunity to practice empathy. "What is this person feeling? How would I feel if I were in his shoes?" And also, "Ultimately, what is the root of this person's problem?"

Give the patient the benefit of the doubt – they may just be having a bad day. Sitting in a packed waiting room, feeling sick and miserable can be enough to make even the most mentally stable person act out.

It is also helpful to remind yourself that some patients don't actually want their problems solved. This can be very difficult, especially for newer physicians, to accept. Why would someone come to the office if not for our advice or treatment recommendations?

It may seem strange to us, but sometimes all that a person wants is to be heard, to vent or to be validated. Even when our patients choose not to make any changes in their lifestyle or health regimen, they may leave the office feeling better just from being listened to.

Often our patients will start to respond to our recommendations after they come to trust us over a series of visits. Having a breakthrough with a challenging patient can be extremely rewarding.

FREQUENT FOLLOW-UP

Frequent follow-up is also very useful for dealing with challenging patients and the cornerstone of treatment of somatoform disorder (see upcoming section).

"Frequent follow up really is the key to dealing with a challenging patient," says Dr. Emily Nabors. In the era of fifteen minute visits (or less!), it is almost impossible to cover all necessary medical territory in one office visit, even with some of your simplest issues. With a challenging patient, time constraints are compounded.

For nearly every type of challenging patient, frequent follow-up will provide the time that you need to gain patient confidence, allow them to fully express their concerns, and to troubleshoot and prevent unscheduled work-in visits.

This is especially important for helping to win patients over. It may take some time for the patient to warm up to you as their new physician, but after several nonthreatening, nonjudgmental visits she may be more accepting of your advice and recommendations.

When scheduling follow-up appointments, give ranges like 2-4 weeks or 1-2 days. This allows the patient control and helps them to factor in issues like finances, time off from work, and emotional processing. Never be afraid to see the patient back sooner rather than later - many patients, especially those who are challenging, prefer to be seen sooner. Some of the psychological reasons for this (fear of abandonment) are discussed in the section below on "Taking Care of the Hateful Patient."

CONSIDER MENTAL ILLNESS

Patients with mental illness can represent a particular challenge in primary care, especially when they haven't yet been officially "diagnosed."

An estimated *26.2%* of Americans ages 18 and older (one out of four!) suffer from a diagnosable mental disorder in a given year.[73] These mental health issues can range from anxiety (the most common mental health disturbance in the US) or depression to more severe issues like schizophrenia, bipolar disorder or borderline personality disorder.

Acknowledging that mental health problems exist is a fundamental element to coping with challenging personalities. It is far easier to start to work with a patient when you recognize that their behavior is often part of a disease process, rather than the person just being "difficult."

The Rock Star physician is perfectly placed to help make the diagnosis of mental health problems and to set the patient on an effective treatment course.

Dr. Emily Nabors says: "Remember that mentally ill people get sick too. Don't just assume it's in their heads." In fact, persons with serious mental illness tend to be in poorer physical health than persons without mental illness, especially in regard to obesity, heart disease and gastrointestinal disorders, diabetes, HIV, and chronic pulmonary disease. Psychiatric patients tend to be sicker, partially because of lifestyle, medications, higher rates of substance abuse, and poorer health care. [74]

Whenever I work with a patient that I find particularly challenging because of numerous health complaints, I ask myself: "Could this person be depressed?" Depression is a frequent cause of vague complaints like headaches, fatigue, dizziness, and abdominal pain. Adequate treatment of depression with cognitive behavioral therapy or medication will often resolve the physical symptoms.

Anxiety is the most common mental health problem in the United States and the root of a wide array of health complaints. Anxiety disorder is often much easier for the physician to recognize than the patient and helping the patient identify their own anxiety as the cause of medical symptoms can cause an epiphany in the patient. Diagnosing anxiety can also help you to avoid ordering unnecessary tests -- reassurance is often sufficient once you gain the trust of an anxious patient.

Psychological consultation can be incredibly helpful for patients with physical as well as mental illness. While the primary care physician can certainly initiate diagnosis and treatment, a good psychiatrist has additional tools and resources, as well as experience and knowledge. I try very hard to remove the stigma of psychology – "Are you trying to say I'm crazy, doc?" – and I remind my patients that the "Mental Health Parity Act" mandates that insurance companies cover psychological care at the same level as medical care.

To facilitate and encourage psychological care, I have a handout of all mental health specialists in the area, along with websites and resources for obtaining more information. I've been known to give this form out multiple times to the same patient at subsequent visits.

SOMATOFORM DISORDERS – OR "DO YOUR TEETH ITCH?"

Anxiety seems to be the root of somatoform disorder, a challenging condition that causes multiple unexplained physical symptoms.[75] Patients with somatization tend to be very preoccupied with their physical symptoms, despite evidence showing that there is no underlying medical cause. Without an adequate diagnosis, these patients may go from doctor to doctor, repeating unnecessary tests.

Patients with somatoform disorder can be especially stressful for physicians. As physicians we feel rewarded when we solve clinical problems and when we can't do this for the medical complaints of somatoform patients, we become frustrated and disappointed.[76] In fact, when I asked my colleagues what type of patient they found the most difficult, many responded with the same answer: "The Worried Well."

Frustration can be decreased if we learn to identify and diagnose somatization. Using a tool called "emotion-focused interviewing," which involves relating the patient's emotions to their physical symptoms, with anxiety in particular being a major emotional contributor, is very helpful. In other words, what were you feeling when you began to have the stomach ache? What seems to be triggering these headaches? Studies show that emotional stress and unconscious anxiety seem to be the trigger for somatization symptoms, as anxiety leads to "striated and smooth muscle tension," causing multiple physical manifestations.[77]

The Patient Health Questionnaire (PHQ) somatoform screening form can also help to diagnose this disorder.[78] If a patient reports being bothered "a lot" by at least three of the following symptoms (without an adequate medical explanation), somatoform disorder should be considered: stomach pain, back pain, pain in the arms, legs or joints, menstrual cramps, pain or problems during sexual intercourse, headaches, chest pain, dizziness, fainting spells, palpitations, shortness of breath, constipation, loose bowels or diarrhea, nausea, gas or indigestion.

I think that another clue of somatoform disorder is when the patient's allergy list is longer than their medication list. This is usually a sign that the patient has been prescribed multiple medications in an attempt to treat these vague symptoms, with various "reactions" to these medications.

Treatment of somatization involves helping the patient to understand that there isn't anything seriously wrong with their health, getting him to psychiatric care (if accepted by the patient) and as always, a schedule of regular, brief follow-up office visits with the physician.

"The first thing that I do with a somatoform patient is to acknowledge that the fact that they really have this and thank heavens, there isn't something structurally wrong," says Dr. Douglas Meuser. "Instead of saying that a work-up is negative, I say that the work-up is 'nondiagnostic,' and fortunately the evaluation doesn't require surgery – 'isn't that great?' I try to stay positive."

Psychiatric consultation is effective in treating patients with somatoform disorder,[79] with even a *single* visit to a psychiatrist showing improvement in patient physical functioning and decreased health care costs.[80]

Other interventions found to be beneficial in treating somatoform disorder include antidepressants, cognitive-behavioral therapy, and group therapy. Cognitive behavioral therapy seems to be the most beneficial treatment.[81]   As with depression and anxiety, diagnosing and treating somatization can resolve many of the physical symptoms, preventing unnecessary testing, and decreasing stress on the patient and physician.

CHRONIC NON-MALIGNANT PAIN SYNDROMES

Many physicians find patients with chronic pain to be very stressful, but there are tools that the Rock Star physician can use to help manage pain.

"Acknowledge pain – pain is real," says Dr. Doug Meuser.   "Most people think of pain as damage – 'I can't have pain, pain is bad.' Once I have ruled out a truly structural problem, I can put someone at ease by acknowledging the fact that their subjective issues are very real but have no structural basis.   Patients are often afraid that they will damage themselves – they will even stop their lives. I try to tell them 'here's what you *can* do.'"

Dr. Meuser suggests helping patients reflect on what pain means to them. "I try to look at the data objectively and help them with their struggle; give them new paths that they haven't imagined. Sometimes you can get to the point where you can look at the patient and say 'you're just going to have to suck it up and get moving.'"

Having a script or structured approach to patients with chronic pain is essential. Standardized forms and checklists can be very beneficial, with tools available from many Pain Management sites. "I have a script that takes me away from the secondary gain that can sometimes occur with chronic pain," says Dr. Meuser. "Taking the emotion out and not getting overinvolved with the patient's situation is essential. If I engage in the patient at their level, I will only see what they want me to see."

And as always, frequent follow-up. "I always leave the patient with the knowledge that they are always welcome back. It may be the end of the 'act' but it's not the end of the play."

THE PROBLEM OF FATIGUE

"Doctor, why am I *so* tired all the time?" Ugh. I'm tired just listening to the question.

About 20% of the general population reports substantial fatigue lasting six months or longer, with women more likely to report fatigue than men.[82] In a primary care setting, the rate of fatigue was found to be even higher at 27%,[83] with little improvement at one-year follow-up.[84] When compared with those reporting no fatigue, people with fatigue were significantly more likely to have experienced depression, anxiety, panic disorder, and somatization disorder, including medically unexplained physical symptoms and increased medical utilization.[85]

Well, I could have told you that!

Here's the deal. Only 15% of patients in primary care are found to have an organic cause for their fatigue, and laboratory testing has not been shown to be very useful in determining an underlying cause. [86]

I like to focus on the practical: What time do you go to bed and get up? Do you sleep well? Do you eat healthily? Do you exercise? No, no, and no? Hmm…

So, I guess on the positive side, we can reassure ourselves (and our patients), that fatigue is common and unlikely to be anything "serious." We can treat any underlying psychological conditions and continue to practice, practice, and practice our attitude of empathy.

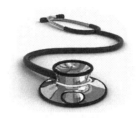

CHAPTER THIRTY-THREE
MANAGING THE CHALLENGING PATIENT

AVOIDING JUDGMENT

One of the very important clinical skills of a Rock Star physician is making a quick diagnostic assessment of a patient. While the initial impression of a patient can provide important clues for diagnosing illness, quick judgment can be tricky in dealing with the challenging patient.

A person having a bad day (or week or month) will often give an inaccurate impression of their true personality or character. So will feeling sick, nauseated, depressed, anxious or in pain.

One strategy to coping with a patient having a bad day is to ask yourself: "What would I feel like if I were having the same problem?" Or even better, "What must it be like to be you?" Essentially, this is *empathy* or "feeling" someone else's pain. We may not be able to actually experience empathy all the time, but we can practice the technique of empathetic thinking.

"It is very important for physicians to be careful about not allowing patients to blame themselves for their health issues," says Dr. Doug Meuser.

It's also important to be nice. I'll never forget the patient who returned to my office for several weeks with vague complaints of "just not feeling right." After a thorough medical evaluation and attempts at treating possible underlying depression, I was getting frustrated. It was on the tip of my tongue to snap at this patient, when a little voice inside stopped me, and instead I said, "I'm sorry that I don't know what's wrong with you, but we're going to keep looking until we find out." A few days later the patient had a seizure and a CT scan in the emergency department revealed a malignant brain tumor. Diagnosing the tumor a few weeks earlier wouldn't have changed the prognosis, but I'm sure the patient and family would have remembered my harsh words if I'd said them.

USE VALIDATION AND CLARIFICATION OF EMOTIONS

One way of practicing empathy is to use a modeling or validating technique. Repeating a patient's words, validating the emotion, and clarifying their feelings can defuse the most stressful situation. Example: Patient has been waiting an hour to see you. You enter the room with your usual smile and friendly attitude, to be hit immediately with a glare and an angry "I've been waiting an hour!" Despite your apology and attempts to placate the patient, she continues to present an angry affect, arms crossed in front of her. "Someone should have told me how late you were. Now I'm going to be late to work!" The atmosphere is tense. Your immediate internal reaction is annoyance and maybe even a little anger. You're running late because you had to give bad news to another patient. Or maybe you had to call 911 for a walk-in patient with chest pain. Maybe you missed lunch, and you're a little cranky.

Stop.

Countering a patient's negative attitude with your own will fail every time. At this moment, the patient doesn't really care about your situation. She is anxious and upset because she is going to be late. Maybe she's been reprimanded about being late in the past and is going to get into trouble when she gets to work. Or maybe she's just upset and wants to express her emotion. This is the perfect opportunity to defuse a negative situation with the validation and clarification method.

"It sounds like you are really stressed about getting to work late." *Repeat the patient's words and express the emotion in neutral terms.* "Is that right?" *Clarify the emotion.* This gets the patient to agree with you and you start on common ground.

"I know that I would be really upset if I were kept waiting so long." *Validate the emotion.*

The patient may agree with your assessment: "Well, yes... but I suppose it will be ok now that you're here... "Or the patient may disagree with your expression. "No, it's not really that I'm going to be late. It's just that I'm worried about my test results."

Generally the patient wants to move forward, but gets stuck on the negative emotion. Validating and clarifying the emotion blocks negative energy from spiraling out of control. It also helps you to understand what the patient is *really* concerned about.

BEWARE OF COUNTERTRANSFERENCE

It's also really important not to allow a person's "issues" to transfer onto you. The term countertransference refers to the response elicited in a therapist (or physician) from the patient's transference. In other words, the patient unconsciously projects or transfers feelings from a previous or current relationship onto the physician, which in turn can create a negative or maladaptive reaction by the physician back onto patient. Confused yet?

Understanding your own emotional reaction to your patients can help create immunity to negative feelings. If you feel yourself becoming stressed, angry, confused (or even murderous, according to studies!) during an interaction with a patient, stop and reflect that these emotions are being elicited in response to the patient's psychological problems, not yours.

If you are still struggling with strong emotions – and psychiatrists warn that "some patients have a powerful ability to project painful states of mind into the people who treat them" – consider using a trained psychologist to help you understand your own "unconscious needs and fears."[87] Yeah, you've got some.

DEALING WITH POOR COMMUNICATORS

THE TALKER

Bottom line: Try not to interrupt. Oh, it's hard, really hard. But ultimately, if you stop the flow, you will just make it worse on yourself. Now you got the talker off subject and he will find a way to get back to the previous discussion, probably starting over from the beginning. Talkers tend to get frustrated when they get off-track and really need to feel that they have been heard. Interestingly, talkers don't require as much active listening. One of the characteristics of the talker is that they will continue on and on, even when you give them little feedback. A way of coping with a talker is to work on your charting while you listen with half an ear for them to wrap up their train of thought. Another way of redirecting is to stand up and start doing a basic examination as the patient continues talking. Once the talker takes a breath, you can usually redirect the conversation.

Dr. Emily Nabors prearranges her nurse to interrupt her on her more talkative patients. "I have the nurse knock on the door after a reasonable amount of time to tell me that I have patients waiting. This takes the pressure off of me. 'I'm sorry I don't have more time, but we can pick this up next week.'"

THE TANGENT

The tangent skips from subject to subject in a stream of consciousness sort of pattern. Keeping conversations on track is critical to increasing efficiency and maximizing physician time.[88]

This can be really tough as a physician attempts to query the patient on symptoms to try to formulate a working diagnosis. Unlike the talker, the tangent can usually be safely interrupted, as they are comfortable skipping around topics. Use the power of redirection, by politely interrupting, returning the conversation back to the subject of interest. Use nonverbal cues like standing or putting your hand up. Acknowledge the digression – "I know you're worried about your cats, but I need to know more about…" You might have to do this repeatedly.

THE STOIC

The perfect example of a stoic patient is the teenager that was dragged in by mom or dad. They tend to respond with shrugs, blank stares, and one-word answers when pressed. The stoic will make you earn your money by dragging the history out of them tooth and nail. Often stoics have a lot of insecurity and anxiety. Be patient. It generally takes several visits for the stoic to gain confidence and warm up to the physician.

WORKING WITH EXTREMELY ILL PEOPLE

Interestingly, many extremely ill people don't really realize how sick they really are. I'm constantly meeting patients who tell me, "Don't worry, you won't have any trouble with me, I'm really healthy." Meanwhile, I'm staring at a list of 20-odd medications, multiple lab abnormalities, and life-threatening chronic conditions. The same goes for geriatric patients - I've learned that many 70- and even 80-year old patients consider themselves in "excellent" health and that in their mind, they are that same healthy 30-year old.

I used to feel quite anxious when I would see a patient with a long list of medical problems or significantly advanced age - 90 year olds are not uncommon in my south Florida area. Ultimately though, I've realized that extremely sick individuals are sometimes easier to work with than those who have never had any medical interactions. Patients with chronic health issues are used to having doctor visits, understand the importance of follow-up and taking medications as prescribed, and often don't see even major medical diagnoses as more than just another hurdle to jump over.

On the flip side, a very healthy person with no previous medical interactions, will sometimes have an emotional melt-down over something as medically basic as a common cold or relatively easily treated as migraine headaches. This type of patient can take a significant amount of physician energy to cope with the problem.

DIAGNOSTIC DILEMMAS

Every physician has that one complaint or symptom that elicits the "groan" response. I would say that mine is dizziness. The differential diagnosis is just so extensive - ranging from the most benign cause like an inner ear viral infection to the most serious pathology like a brain tumor or potentially lethal cardiac arrhythmia.

I don't love it when I see dizziness on the chief complaint, but I don't fear it. Why? Because I've prepared a script for dealing with my most challenging medical diagnoses so that I can formulate a treatment plan in a coherent and logical way, and I also keep in mind that fact that many challenging diagnoses are mimics of mental disorders like depression, anxiety, and somatization.

Dr. Doug Meuser calls this kind of script: "Taking the hate out of ___ (fill in the blank with your particular diagnosis of loathing)." "I use a structured approach to look at all of the data in an objective way."

One of the best ways to achieve this is to create a customized template incorporating a typical history and physical within a particular differential diagnosis. For example, your dizziness template will take you through common neurologic, cardiac, ENT, and psychiatric historical elements. If your template is very clear, you can even have your medical assistant start to question the patient and enter some of the data into the medical record before you see the patient.

A template examination section will pre-populate your standard detailed ENT, neurologic and cardiac examination, which you can edit as appropriate. And your assessment/plan section will include your usual differential diagnosis for dizziness, with the appropriate work-up for the diagnoses you think most likely based on the history and physical.

Also helping my attitude in dealing with diagnostic dilemmas is the realization that any such complaint is an automatic "level 5" visit- in other words, the highest paying code, because it is going to require an extensive evaluation and management plan and if you have to consider life-threatening causes, this is a high-risk scenario.

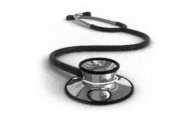

CHAPTER THIRTY-FOUR
THE TRULY HATEFUL PATIENT

James Groves, MD, wrote a wonderful article in 1978 called "Taking Care of the Hateful Patient,"[89] which I think should be recommended reading for all physicians. The hateful patient is someone that elicits an extreme reaction in physicians - "fear, despair, and even malice."

Dr. Groves breaks down the most challenging patients into four main categories, and interestingly the bottom line for managing all four types comes down to *validating concerns and frequent follow-up.*

See if you recognize any of these patients in your practice.

The **"dependent clinger"** is exhaustingly needy. These patients tend to call often and drop by the office without appointments, but are usually not aware of the negative effect that they are having on the physician. They easily feel rejected.

It's important to recognize this type of patient early on in your encounters with him. Common signs are excessive compliments -"You saved my life!" when you really just prescribed an antibiotic, or, "You're the *best* doctor I have ever had!" when he only met you once. Our natural inclination is to be flattered by these types of patients, but don't get too excited - soon enough the situation will escalate from one of pleasantries to that of a nuisance, as the patient drops by or calls more and more often for nothing in particular.

According to Dr. Groves, the best way to work with the dependent clinger is to "tactfully and firmly" explain to the patient that you as a physician have limits, and schedule routine follow up visits with reminders not to call except during office hours or in an emergency.

The "**entitled demander**" is needy, but unlike the clinger, he *is* aware of the effect that he has on the physician, and may use "intimidation, devaluation, and guilt induction." Dr. Groves points out that these patients don't realize that it is their own "deep dependency and terror of abandonment" that trigger their behaviors.

When you meet a patient like this, you will often feel fearful and an inclination towards "counterattack," but the best technique is to acknowledge the patient's entitlement, and "rechannel it" in a more productive way, by agreeing that the patient *is* entitled - not to unreasonable demands or bullying, but to the best medical care possible. Dr. Groves says that there should be "tireless repetition" in validating that the patient indeed deserves 'first-rate' medical care.

The "**manipulative help-rejecter**" never seems to get better, no matter what treatment the physician offers. Even if one symptom is improved, another "mysteriously appears in its place." This is a somatoform type patient in the extreme. After initial anxiety in the physician ("did I miss something?"), the doctor generally becomes irritable and depressed, feeling guilty and inadequate. Dr. Groves points out that the help-rejecter usually is depressed himself, although he tends to deny depression and refuse referral to psychology. A way to manage this patient is to "share the pessimism by saying that treatment may not be entirely curative," but to schedule routine follow-up, which keeps the patient from feeling abandoned.

Finally, the **"self-destructive denier"** displays "unconsciously self-murdering behaviors, which may be a chronic form of suicidal behavior; often they let themselves die." Dr. Groves says that these patients are the hardest to help. We need to recognize that these patients may provoke strong feelings, such as malice and "the fervent wish that they would die and 'get it over with.'" Accepting that these emotions are normal will keep the physician from abandoning the patient. A psychiatric consultation may be able to help, but the self-destructive denier usually refuses, as with other treatment options.

Ultimately, as doctors we have to understand and accept the emotions that challenging patients provoke. To deny our own feelings can lead to errors in diagnosis and treatment, as well as damage our own psyche.

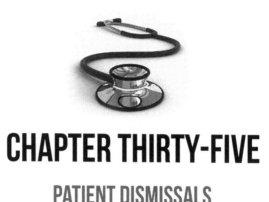

CHAPTER THIRTY-FIVE
PATIENT DISMISSALS

Sometimes the best way to deal with a challenging patient is to dismiss them from your practice. Drastic, yes, but sometimes it is absolutely necessary.

- **Frequent no-shows**. Patients that repeatedly miss appointments are a source of lost revenue, take up space in the schedule that other patients could use, and are a set up for liability in the case of poor health outcomes. Always document no-shows by generating a no-show letter. And have an office policy for dismissal after a certain number of missed appointments.

- **Extreme noncompliance**. We've discussed the management of the noncompliant patient in detail. Sometimes regardless of your best efforts, a patient will continue to decline your recommendations so that the consequences create a hardship not only for that person, but for you and your office staff. For example, I finally dismissed a hard-smoking, hard-drinking, brittle diabetic, severely hypertensive man with known coronary disease after multiple walk-ins to the office requiring me to call 911. Upon return from the hospital we would talk about him taking his medications and quitting smoking. He would agree - and then a few weeks later he would be back in my office, off of his medications, and again in an emergency state - usually chest pain or shortness of breath. Every time this happened, my office schedule would be thrown into disarray as I dealt with his emergency and shipped him off to the hospital. It wasn't fair to me, to my other patients or to my staff. After advising him that if he continued to smoke and not take his medications, I would not be able to see him back in the practice, I finally sent him a letter of dismissal. Interestingly, a year or two later he showed up in my office just to say 'hi' and to let me know that he had quit smoking.

- **Threats/verbal abuse/mean people**. Everyone has a bad day every now and then. An occasional sharp tone of voice, a frustrated expression of discontent - understandable. But verbal abuse, cursing, shouting, and threats are not tolerated in my office, whether they are focused at me or at any of my staff members. Also, patient threats of "Fine, then I'll just find another doctor!" are met with an immediate termination letter from the practice - "I understand that you are electing to find another physician. This letter is to acknowledge that the physician-patient relationship has been terminated and that Dr. B will no longer be responsible for your care."

- **You've just had enough**. There is occasionally a patient that will just push your buttons. Without being able to reconcile the emotions that the patient arouses in you, you are not going to be

214

able to provide the patient with the best care that they deserve, and you are going to make yourself crazy. Dismiss.

WHEN A PATIENT THREATENS YOU

To be threatened by a patient is a very scary situation for a physician. Unfortunately, the reality is that physicians have been injured and even killed by disgruntled patients so threats or other warning signs of violence should be taken very seriously.

Contact your local Sheriff Department immediately for threats against yourself or your office staff. Your office should have a policy on handling threats or violence in the practice. It's always a good policy to keep patient care areas locked to prevent anyone from walking in. Panic-buttons or alarms can be installed at the front desk to contact local police in case of an emergency situation.

I have been threatened by several patients, each of whom had underlying mental illness. One of these patients, a young man with brain damage from an auto accident, told his physical therapist "I'm going to get a gun, go to Dr. Bernard's office and kill her" because I wouldn't authorize the return of his drivers' license.

A visit from a Sheriff's deputy and trip to our local psychiatric crisis unit prevented the situation from escalating, but I won't deny that I was frightened and anxious.

THE TERMINATION LETTER

Ending a physician-patient relationship requires care and tact. As a non-confrontational physician, I prefer to notify my patients in writing rather than in person, although other physicians choose to give the news directly.

Carlos Portu, MD, avoids dismissing patients whenever possible, but when it has to be done, he is direct. "I have forgiven patients for being rude and throwing a fit, but what I don't like is if I'm in the room with someone and they've made it clear that they're unhappy to be there, displeased with me, and don't want to hear what I am telling them. I'm quite frank with them – 'you need to be at the place where you feel comfortable, and that may not be here.'"

"Dismissing a patient isn't a confrontation, it's a decision that has already been made," says Douglas Meuser, MD. "I don't engage, I just say 'it's not working out.' That takes the emotion out of it."

There are steps to take when dismissing a patient that will protect the physician from an accusation of patient abandonment. In general, the American Medical Association (AMA) recommends giving 30 days notice, during which you will provide emergency medical care. Send this notice by certified mail, advising the patient of the need to find another physician immediately, and providing information on how to obtain a copy of the medical records. Keep this dismissal letter in the patient's chart.

SAMPLE DISMISSAL LETTER

Dear _____:

I find it necessary to inform you that I will no longer be able to serve as your physician. The physician/patient relationship is extremely important to your health and well-being, and I do not believe that our relationship is effective. Our relationship has been damaged because {reason for discharge -- for example, not compliant, missing appointments, not following treatment recommendations}.

I recommend you promptly find another physician to provide your medical care. The county medical society can provide you with a list of physicians in the area.

I will be available to treat you on an emergency basis only until {30 days from date of letter}. This will give you time to find a new physician. Enclosed is an authorization form that permits me to send your new physician a copy of your medical records.

Sincerely,

ROCK STAR MD/ DO

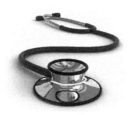

CHAPTER THIRTY-SIX

DEATH AND DYING – THE TERMINALLY ILL PATIENT

We couldn't end our discussion of challenging clinical issues without discussing death and dying, an integral aspect of all medical practice. As physicians, we have to accept and cope with the inevitable nature of death, both in our own mortality and that of our patients. We have to learn to give painful news to patients and to their loved ones. We also have to learn the tools that we need to help ease suffering and provide quality end-of-life care. None of these elements are easy, but they are an essential responsibility of a physician.

My experience with death and dying as a medical student was limited to one week of in-patient hospice shadowing, as well as the deaths of critically ill hospital patients, most of whom I knew only superficially. In residency, I gained little more experience in the dying process, usually amounting to giving bad news in the hospital setting, usually after a code blue, and always with a fellow resident.

Outside of the hospital, my entire experience with death and dying was in caring for one personal clinic patient, a young woman who suffered a remission of melanoma and died during my final year of training. I followed her with the hospice team, even paying a home visit with a hospice nurse, who was stunned that a doctor wanted to participate in the process. Although I did very little to help my patient, after she died her partner sent me a beautiful note telling me how much it meant that I was there for Judy during her last weeks.

Aside from this experience with hospice, I had little knowledge or insight into the dying process. A personal experience taught me how little I really knew: Upon visiting my grandmother with end-stage COPD, she developed a severe flare up. She had classic "air hunger," gasping for breath, eyes bulging, blue lips – but adamantly refused to let us call 911 or take her to the hospital. After multiple hospital admissions involving painful blood tests and near intubation, she had had enough. "No more," she gasped, shaking her head adamantly.

I was just 4 months into my intern year. All I knew about COPD at that time involved aggressive care – so I tried what I could. I gave her a nebulized breathing treatment. I got her to swallow a few tablets of prednisone. And I watched her die, helpless to alleviate her suffering.

If I had only known then that all I had to do was to pick up the phone and call the local hospice. A hospice nurse would have come over with a "comfort care kit" - a little morphine to stop the sensation of suffocation, an anxiety medicine to help her relax, as well as oxygen and a fan to blow on her to comfort her breathing. It didn't have to happen that way.

END-OF-LIFE CARE

Being there for our patients at the end of life and giving them "permission" to stop futile aggressive interventions is one of the greatest gifts that we can give our patients. It is our job to be honest with our patients, avoiding false hope for survival, but instead focusing on a "good death." We have to be the ones to give the hard facts – that feeding tubes don't improve quality of life in end-stage dementia, but grandpa isn't going to experience hunger or thirst. And to share that chemotherapy in advanced metastatic cancer won't prolong life, and choosing not to accept it is not "giving up."

It is amazing and sad how many patients are compelled into accepting painful time-consuming treatments due to pressure from physicians and family members.

Not only can these procedures be uncomfortable and futile, but they also cut into time that could be spent doing other activities like spending time with family or traveling while they are still well enough to do it.

Sometimes patients just need to hear that it's OK to say "no," and that you will be on their side and support them no matter what.

Patients facing the end of life are often afraid, not always of the finality of death, but of pain, of being alone or being abandoned. We must assure them that we will continue to provide them medical care – but for comfort, rather than for cure.

So, when is it the right time to bring up the "H-word:" Hospice?

The medical criterion for hospice admission is a life expectancy of six months or less. So if you would be surprised to hear that your patient was alive in six months, then that person is a potential candidate.

I like to bring up the topic if my patient expresses the desire to avoid future hospitalization. A comment like "I'm never going back there" is an opportunity to educate your patient on the hospice option. This way the patient and family will avoid the fear and anxiety of coping with acute symptoms at home – which often results in a 911 call if the patient and family panic.

Unfortunately, an ambulance transfer to the ER will often lead to unwanted aggressive treatment, sometimes despite a DNR being present. Instead, if a patient has discomfort, hospice can be contacted to treat symptoms and avoid the hospital.

It's so important to address hospice *before* such a crisis occurs. Our job is to help patients understand that choosing hospice does not mean that they, or we, are giving up, but rather that we are changing the goals of therapy to comfort rather than cure.

Family members often experience severe guilt – "am I doing the right thing?" – when deciding on end-of-life issues, like stopping life support or even transferring a loved one into a hospice facility in the final days of life. Our job as their physician is to support families in these decisions, to guide them, and to reassure them that what they are doing is in the best interest of the patient.

Dr. Ariel Cole, a Geriatrician in Orlando, Florida, tells her patients: "I may not have a cure for your disease, but I will walk this road with you."

Sometimes, that is enough.

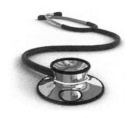

CHAPTER THIRTY-SEVEN

FINDING THE ANSWERS

According to Malcolm Gladwell's book "Outliers," it takes at least 10,000 hours to develop expertise in a subject.[90] Well guess what – we've already doubled that by the time we graduate residency. The American Academy of Family Physicians (AAFP) estimates that the average family doctor graduates with 21,000 total hours of training.[91]

But those 21,000 hours are just getting us started! Once we graduate from residency, where we had professors and colleagues to consult with, we are officially "on our own," where we face another sharp learning curve, and probably at least another 10,000 hours of practice to hone our skills.

The good news is that we don't have to know all the answers. In fact, it's impossible to know all the answers, especially with constant updates and scientific breakthroughs. However, *we do* have to know where to find the answers and to find them quickly and efficiently in a way that maximizes patient-physician face-to-face time.

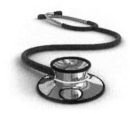

CHAPTER THIRTY-EIGHT
USING EVIDENCE-BASED MEDICINE (EBM)

Evidence based medicine was just in its infancy as I was graduating from medical school. In fact, I remember back then that many physicians resented the idea of EBM – seeing it as an algorithmic debasement of the physician experience and the art of medicine.

At this point, most physicians have embraced the idea of EBM, while recognizing that the science of medicine is constantly evolving, as studies confirm or refute formerly held ideas.

For example, my final exam in my Family Medicine rotation in medical school involved me explaining to a mock patient how important it was to start her on hormone replacement therapy (HRT) after menopause. I remember telling her all the wonderful benefits, from osteoporosis prevention to improved quality of life. To have failed to convince the patient would have resulted in a failing grade.

Fast-forward just three years later, as the Women's Health Initiative (WHI) study blew the lid off of the HRT movement, showing that rather than benefiting women, HRT actually increased the risk of heart attacks and strokes!

I can even remember where I was when I heard that news – sitting in a hotel lobby while CNN reported on the study. I was completely floored – my world was rocked, everything I had believed and convinced patients to believe was wrong. And it left me somewhat stunned.

While my response might seem a bit melodramatic, this was my first true experience with evidence-based medicine, and the power of it was profound.

Although certainly much of medicine lacks good evidence or scientific research, when there is evidence to support or refute a given treatment, the Rock Star doctor is ready to consider the data and evolve his practice in response. He might even go so far as to quip: "In God we trust; all others must bring (randomized, double-blinded, controlled) data."

I like to joke with my patients: "This is what the current guidelines say – when they change I'll let you know." Another good reason for regular follow-up!

An excellent source for good evidence-based medicine is the Cochrane Library, a collection of database meta-analyses. Other sources include the website www.guideline.gov, as well as numerous other websites and journals emphasizing EMB.

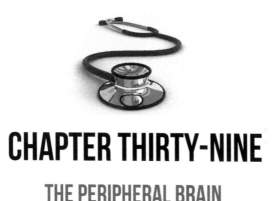

CHAPTER THIRTY-NINE

THE PERIPHERAL BRAIN

While we don't have to know all of the answers, we do have to know where to find them. The best source: medical literature. Remember the days when you had to spend hours in the medical library searching through giant textbooks or in the basement "stacks" reviewing journal articles?

No? Lucky you.

In the Internet age, the answers are literally at our fingertips via web searches, <u>PubMed</u> and <u>Medline</u> reviews, and resources like <u>Epocrates</u> and <u>Medscape</u>. Many of these resources are available on tablet and smart-phones.

No more rushing out of the exam room to dig through your massive "Cecil's Textbook of Medicine" index for several year old data! Now we can just pull out our tablet computer and have a current answer within seconds. Dr. Jennifer Keehbauch keeps her iPhone in the office with her, so that she can immediately pull up resources. "I also write myself little notes in my phone to remember specific protocols or medication dosing."

While there are many wonderful websites, my very favorite is <u>Up-to-Date</u>. Almost every doctor I polled agreed that Up-to-Date was their "go-to" site for medical guidance. This resource provides a comprehensive review of medical topics, with an emphasis on evidence, but also incorporating expert-based opinion where firm data is lacking. Each article has links to other related topics, and physicians can use this information to guide evaluation and treatment options, even printing out patient education resources from the site. And no, I am not a paid sponsor for Up-To-Date.

I also enjoy subscribing to <u>"Prescriber's Letter</u> – Unbiased Recommendations You Can Trust on New Developments in Drug Therapy." This is a monthly newsletter with the latest evidence-based information on medications, and one of the few medical subscriptions that I actually pay for.

BRINGING THE PERIPHERAL BRAIN INTO THE EXAM ROOM

Guess what? It's OK to look up information in front of your patient. It's always better to look something up than to make a guess leading to an incorrect diagnosis or treatment. In general, your patients will not think less of you – and believe it or not, some patients actually like it: "Wow, my doctor really wants to makes sure he is doing the best thing for me!"

As David Voran, MD, recommends, "Never leave the room to look up something … use your computer to Google, UpToDate or ZygoteBody the answers and bring the patients along in the learning."

Because science always changes and evolves, none of us can always stay current on every topic. Sometimes I pull open a medical website just to make sure that nothing new has popped up on a tough illness to treat or to confirm a medication dose that I haven't prescribed for a while. I also use non-medical websites – Google Images is one of my favorite resources for showing pictures of the human body and various disease processes.

Dr. Doug Meuser uses a small tablet computer to bring up resources in the exam room with the patient. "This is the beauty of informatics to engage the patient in their own care. We can enter information together, and we are both focused on the information. I tell them: this is not just my opinion, it's guidance from somebody a whole lot smarter."

I also love to use the Internet for patient-focused sources like insurance formularies, locating specialists, and pricing databases (www.goodrx. com is a great site to check medication costs for cash-paying patients).

The Rock Star doctor should have Internet access in every room, so that she can pull up helpful resources instantly. If you're anything like me, by the time you get into your office you may forget what you were going to look up.

THE SCIENTIFIC "TOOLS OF THE TRADE"

Like scientific calculators replacing the slide rule, the Internet has revolutionized the use of medical calculations and algorithms.

These web-based tools allow physicians to quickly calculate and assess important details like the risk of heart attacks, strokes, pulmonary emboli, and osteoporotic fractures. They help us and our patients to weigh the risks and benefits before using medications.

We can calculate a person's kidney and liver function, determine the risk of Tylenol toxicity, and decide when an x-ray of the ankle or knee is indicated. The website www.mdcalc.com is an excellent resource, and Jennifer Keehbauch, MD, loves the app QxCalculate for medical calculations.

Rather than having to retain all of this complicated information in your memory, an unlikely possibility at the best of times, the Rock Star physician can access what Dr. Doug Meuser calls his "peripheral brain" at any time. Not only can these resources provide vital information, but they can also be used to educate patients about their own health.

USING TOOLS FOR PATIENT CARE

In the hospital, most medical calculations are used to dose medication correctly or to make a quick diagnosis like evaluating for a pulmonary embolus. In primary care, my most useful scientific tools allow me to help my patients understand more about their own health risks and benefits to using medications.

For example, I love to use the Framingham Risk Assessment to help patients determine whether or not a statin drug to lower their cholesterol would be beneficial. After entering the patient's data into the chart and determining the 10-year heart attack risk, we can then go back into the calculator model, changing just the cholesterol number to what we might expect if we used a statin drug. The change in cardiac risk can be very compelling to help a patient understand the potential benefit of using a statin drug.

On the other hand, sometimes the risk reduction is so small that a patient may elect *not* to use a statin medication. But the bottom line is that they now have a measure to help with educated, meaningful decision making.

Another great calculation is the FORE (Foundation for Osteoporosis Education) score to determine the risk of osteoporosis related fractures. Seeing the fracture risk can help a patient decide if the benefits of taking medication outweigh the potential risks.

Scientific evidence is constantly helping to develop and revise new calculator models to help predict disease and evaluate treatment options. Using this data, the physician can create personalized medicine and really be a Rock Star.

THE LIABILITIES OF EVIDENCE-BASED MEDICINE (EBM)

EBM is far from perfect. First of all, there just isn't good data for a lot of medical issues. Secondly, not everyone "fits the mold" – some people, despite the "evidence," may not be good candidates for certain medical treatments based on other health issues, may choose not to follow guidelines for various reasons or don't respond to the recommended, evidence-based treatment plan.

This is where we can argue against what some call cookie-cutter medicine. Medicine is *not* one-size-fits-all, the algorithms don't work for everyone, and there is definitely an art as well as science to medicine.

Finally, the evidence is constantly in flux. What was once conventional wisdom may now be considered a complete fallacy. Yesterday, everyone was on fish oil and calcium. Today we say these supplements are a waste of money. And tomorrow? Who knows?

Sometimes a physician's personal experience with a treatment plan will serve him better than current guidelines. There are times when listening to that "little voice inside," although contrary to current guidelines, will serve her better than strict adherence to a particular algorithm. Ultimately, the Rock Star physician has to focus on the patient relationship first and foremost, utilizing EBM whenever possible without becoming stymied by it.

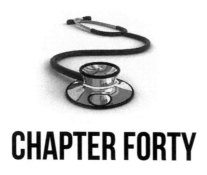

CHAPTER FORTY

FINDING THE ANSWERS:

LABORATORY AND RADIOLOGY TESTING

"Every doctor deserves the results of the tests she ordered." Clichéd, but oh, how true.

Don't get me wrong: I love ordering blood tests. Patients love to have their blood checked. I love to find out the secrets that the blood work gives up. The thrill of finding a low thyroid or a vitamin B12 deficiency – something treatable!

However, blood work needs to be ordered for a specific reason, looking for a particular problem. Fatigued? By all means, let's check blood counts, chemistries, and thyroid function.

But ordering a rheumatoid panel for a patient with just a few aches and pains and with no joint swelling or other signs of inflammatory arthritis? Not a good idea.

Besides the expense of unnecessary testing, what are you going to do when you get an unexpected result, like an auto-immune antibody (ANA) test coming back positive? Let's say the results show a low titer, indicating a probable false positive, probably means nothing, but now you have a needlessly worried patient on your hands, resulting in more testing, and adding to cost and anxiety.

The same goes for radiologic testing. Any time we order an imaging test we take risks – like excessive radiation from CT scans or reactions to intravenous contrast material. The Rock Star doctor should carefully weigh the risks and rewards of labs and radiology tests, like medicines, before administering them.

A WORD ABOUT FASTING LIPID PANELS

Why, oh why must we torture our patients? How many studies do we need to confirm that fasting lipid panels are no better than non-fasting?[92]   If you won't believe the doctors, will you at least believe a nursing study that concludes the same results? [93] And *why* does the lab send my patients away even when their lab slip says, "*Fasting not required?*" We need to make testing easier and rather than more difficult. Not starving our patients is a great way to start.

TREAT THE PATIENT, NOT THE TEST -- OR: DON'T GET SICK IN JULY

In my intern year I learned this lesson the hard way. It was 3 AM; I was covering the entire hospital and the emergency room and had just fallen asleep when my pager rang out. "I have a patient with a hemoglobin of 6," the nurse reported. Groggily I ordered 2 units of packed red blood cells and serial "H and H's" (hemoglobin and hematocrits). A few hours later the nurse called me with the result of my first H/H: Hemoglobin 11.

My heart stopped. There was no way that two units of blood could raise hemoglobin from 6 to 11. I had unnecessarily transfused the patient based on a lab error.

In retrospect, my error was obvious. I had failed to get any history on the patient (any reason to expect bleeding?), I hadn't examined the patient to see if she clinically appeared to be critically anemic; heck, I hadn't even had them re-run a stat hemoglobin to confirm the diagnosis.

As I mentioned in the opening to this book, I've made mistakes and this was the first of many. But I did learn that old but accurate cliché: Treat the patient and not the lab result.

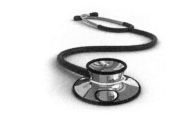

CHAPTER FORTY-ONE
PRACTICE, PRACTICE, PRACTICE

The best tool for patient care is practice. Coming out of residency with our requisite 20,000 + hours still isn't enough. So, how to get that practice when you are first starting out?

I advocate spending a few years after residency working in a high-volume location, ideally with a senior physician on-site or nearby for the occasional curbside consult. One way of achieving this is by working in areas with physician shortages, which is a complete win-win for the new physician as well as patients and communities.

First off, you may be eligible for programs like the <u>National Health Service Corps</u> (NHSC), which provide loan repayment in exchange for a few years of service. Don't forget, you will still be earning a physician's salary as well as the additional loan pay-off. It may not be quite as much as your colleagues will start out with, but the experience will be invaluable. Also, you will likely be protected by sovereign immunity from malpractice suits.

I worked for six years in a Federally Qualified Health Center (FQHC) Health Professional Shortage Area (HPSA) after residency. I called it a second residency, as I think I learned as much in that first year as I did in the rest of my training. Thrown into the fire, I had to care for very sick, uninsured patients without the routine support of attending physicians or subspecialists. I learned how to think outside the box and I spent a ton of time on medical websites strategizing on how best to evaluate various conditions.

I also got to do lots of activities that aren't always possible in conventional private practice - procedures like suturing, removing foreign bodies like fish hooks, and ingrown toenails. I practiced low-risk prenatal care and performed gynecological services like endometrial biopsies and placing intrauterine devices (IUDs).

This setting allowed me to practice the full-spectrum of family medicine - from premature newborn babies, all ages of children, to the most senior of citizens. I treated every type of chronic disease, from diabetes to HIV infection, and managed all sorts of acute illness, from sniffles to anaphylactic reactions. And once I nearly had to deliver a baby in the office. I also supervised a Physician Assistant and several Advanced Practice Nurses, something I never experienced in my residency.

Fortunately, I did have support from several other physicians working at the site, which was really helpful in gaining confidence, especially since the local ambulance was 45 minutes away in the event of an emergency – which happened routinely. Amazingly, after a few years, I became the mentor for new arriving physicians!

As Carrie Gittings, MD, another physician with NHSC experience and now the medical director of an underserved clinic says: "Confidence takes time and practice. And willingness to ask docs with more experience when needed."

Dr. Jennifer Keehbauch practiced in a similar high-volume practice setting early in her career: the military. "I spent three years as a general medical officer." At first, she says, "I didn't have a clue, but I read and asked my partners and learned a lot."

Another way to gain experience is to consider moonlighting. Some residencies allow 3rd year students to work at urgent care clinics or physician offices on the weekends. I practiced (literally) at a private physician office doing acute care and at a college health center. Even now, I do a little side work for my local hospice organization to keep my palliative medicine skills up. Volunteer work at a free medical clinic for the homeless or other disadvantaged groups is another great way of gaining experience and confidence with patient care. Jennifer Keehbauch, MD, volunteered at "Healthcare for the Homeless" during her residency. "It inspired me to a lifetime of commitment for the underserved."

No matter how you do it: Practice. Practice. Practice.

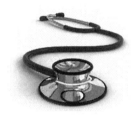

CHAPTER FORTY-TWO

WORKING WITH CONSULTANTS AND THE MEDICAL TEAM

Sometimes despite a primary care doctor's best efforts, it becomes clear that further expertise is needed in diagnosing or treating a condition. A critical skill for a primary care physician is to determine *when* to make the referral and how to communicate with his or her consultants.

A Rock Star physician doesn't just ship patients off to specialists without good reason. In general, primary care docs should have the training to cope with 80-90% of medical problems in the office.

There is a temptation these days as we see more complex patients in shorter visit times, to turf a patient with diabetes, hypertension, and high cholesterol off to an endocrinologist, nephrologist, and cardiologist. While it may initially seem easier to send your patient off to a multitude of other physicians, ultimately this type of referral practice leads to fragmented care, duplicate testing and essentially *more* work as you unravel the care plan initiated by several other doctors.

I've even worked in environments when my consulting specialists have referred my patients to other specialists, bypassing me as the primary care physician. "Hmm, I see that you have checked 'frequent urination' on your form – I'll have you see my Urology colleague. And we'd better get you into Podiatry for that foot pain you mentioned." I call this a pinball machine referral practice, and I don't think it serves patients well.

It is the primary care physician's responsibility to refer only when clinically necessary and to be prompt in referring when it is indicated. The Rock Star physician understands her limitations or, in other words, "knows what she doesn't know" and doesn't let ego get into the way of an appropriate referral.

CHOOSE YOUR CONSULTANTS CAREFULLY

Which would you rather hear: "I loved the doctor you recommended!" or: "That doctor didn't listen to me - why would you send me to her?"

Sounds like a silly question, but this is a scenario that we face in medicine every day. Patients will often judge us by our recommendations, and the Rock Star physician has to consider not only who has the best clinical expertise, but also who has a decent bedside manner and rapport with patients.

Dr. Emily Nabors says, "I refer to doctors that I would go to, or send my family members to. And if I get complaints from my patients, I stop referring there." She also tries to get to know her specialists personally if possible, so that she can call them with questions if necessary. Dr. Roberta Chung also likes to develop a relationship with her colleagues, "If I've got the specialist's cell phone number, it's probably a good sign."

And all the primary care doctors that I spoke to agreed: a note from the specialist in a timely manner is essential.

FACILITATING THE REFERRAL

When I refer a patient to a specialist, I have my office staff help to schedule the appointment and to ensure that the patient has all necessary information – the office phone number, location with map if necessary – and also a copy of their pertinent records to bring to the appointment. Dr. Nabors agrees, "Take care of each referral in-house while the patient is still there."

I also like to send a fax with the patient's information to the consultant - it is critical to provide your consulting physicians with the information that they need to help your patient. The Rock Star doctor will prepare a referral letter describing the reason for referral in detail.

Dear Dr. Neurology Consultant,

Thank you for seeing Mrs. Jones. She has a history of severe migraine headaches despite attempts at treatment with X, Y, and Z. She had a normal MRI in May (attached). I appreciate your evaluation and recommendations for further treatment.

Sincerely,

Rock Star MD/ DO

I always ask my patients to schedule a follow-up appointment with me after they see the consultant. This allows me to find out the patient's understanding of what they were told, so that I can interpret "medical-ese," clarify misunderstandings, and help facilitate the treatment plan and appropriate follow-up.

While the consultant is providing valuable assistance, the primary care physician should be the ultimate facilitator of the patient's care. It is very important that your consultants know that you want to be well informed of any care plan, such as receiving copies of labs and other studies, as well as being notified about upcoming hospitalizations, surgeries or other invasive procedures. We also need to reciprocate by sending our notes and test results to our patients' team of specialists.

The Rock Star physician will make it easy on his consultants - providing the specialist's office with your direct email or cell phone number can be helpful, as well as advising your staff to notify you immediately if another physician is calling.

In my experience, most specialists highly value relationships with primary care physicians – not only as referral sources, but also as members of a health care team.

ROCK STAR REFERRALS - PHYSICAL THERAPY

When I was a third year resident, I went on a mission trip to Mexico. The group included several medical doctors, a group of dentists, and two physical therapists. In my naivety and arrogance as a young physician, I remember asking myself what a Physical Therapist could possibly do to help seriously ill and impoverished people in the small villages that we visited.

After spending hours in a converted schoolhouse doling out multivitamins, de-worming medication, and little packets of Tylenol – about all we could really do with our limited resources – I went outside where I saw an excited group of local people gathered around a man with amputated legs. The physical therapists were designing a custom set of crutches, and the man took his first steps in many years without having to crawl on the ground. His face was beaming with joy as his family members whooped and applauded. The therapists with their skills had changed a life for the better.

Later, I was humbled again as I watched a line of laborers learning stretching exercises to ease their aching necks and backs under the tutelage of the physical therapists. The pain medication I had distributed would soon be gone, but the lessons taught by the therapists could last a lifetime, and could even be taught to others.

A good physical therapist is worth her weight in gold. I keep a list of local therapists and liberally refer my patients with joint pains, muscle spasms, chronic pain, balance issues, weakness, etc. Not only can a physical therapist perform modalities, but he can also give the patient important tools for developing a home exercise program and lifelong healthy practices.

On my referrals, I never condescend to give therapy orders, but rather request, "evaluate and treat." I have long learned that physical therapists know their job far better than I do.

Dr. Doug Meuser, a sports medicine specialist, feels that physical therapy is so important that he developed an in-house physical therapy center at the University of Central Florida Student Health Center. "Get good therapists who see your patients and discharge them – the key is truly focused rehab, with a transition back to the primary care team."

THE HEALTH CARE TEAM

We couldn't care for our patients without a team effort. We need our occupational therapists, speech therapists, case managers and social workers, psychologists, and many other members of the health care team. In fact, on many occasions, I have wished for a good social worker and psychologist to help with the multiple challenges and barriers in obtaining help for patients.

As a physician, I can write prescriptions and referrals all day long, but if the patient can't afford her medications, can't find a ride to the pharmacy or can't read the medication labels, then all my effort is in vain.

A Rock Star physician knows the importance of the health care team and learns to harness these resources. Along with my list of physical therapists, I keep a paper called "Health Care Resources," which includes the phone number and website of various agencies, including governmental, private, and religious organizations – anyone that I think could possibly be able to offer assistance.

Sometimes the hardest place for a patient is to know where to start and just having a phone number can get that person on the right track.

SAMPLE HEALTH CARE RESOURCES FORM

State and County Health Departments
Local Sliding Scale Clinics
Reduced Cost Lab
Women's Health – Planned Parenthood
Health insurance information: www.healthcare.gov
Disability information: www.ssa.gov/pgm/disability.htm
Local/ County Mental Health Centers – Crisis care
Mental Health America – Crisis # 1-800-273-TALK- www.nmha.org
Alcoholics Anonymous
Al-Anon – www.al-anon.org
National Alliance on Mental Illness (NAMI)
Prescription Drug Help:
Partnership for Prescription Assistance -www.pparx.org
Pharmaceutical Assistance programs
Costco, Sam's– may not need membership to use the pharmacy
Publix – Free Lisinopril, Metformin, Amlodipine, and some antibiotics
United Way: 211
Tobacco cessation: Florida Quit line 1-877-U-CAN-NOW
Breast Cancer Susan G Komen- www.komenswfl.org
Local Hospices

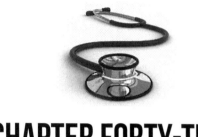

CHAPTER FORTY-THREE
MANAGING HOSPITALIZATIONS

More PCPs are choosing to focus on either in-patient or out-patient medicine exclusively. In fact, the majority of primary care physicians – 67% - (FM, IM, and Peds) spend their time exclusively in the office, relying on hospital-only physicians or hospitalists to manage their patients there.[94]

Many physicians find it unrealistic to practice both in-patient and out-patient medicine, particularly related to balancing work load, such as the burden of traveling for rounds (in my instance, the hospital is a 30-40 minute drive from my office), multiple telephone calls from hospital staff, and less time to focus on out-patient care. In a survey of California Family Physicians, 68% agreed that hospitalists were a "good idea." [95]

On the downside, we may feel that we are abandoning our patients when they feel they need us the most. Hospitalists are not always able to bring the same familiarity and appreciation for the patient's situation as the primary care physician, and we risk communication problems, especially with transition of care upon discharge from the hospital.

The key to Rock Star success when using a hospitalist is developing a follow-up plan to ensure good communication and transition of care back to the outpatient realm.[96] There are three main objectives in sharing care with a hospitalist:

1. We need to know immediately when our patient is admitted to the hospital so that we may provide relevant information to the hospitalist.

2. We need to know promptly when our patient is discharged to ensure a follow-up visit.

3. We need hospital records so that we can appropriately follow up on the care plan.

HOSPITAL ADMISSIONS

Ideally, your local emergency departments should have a system in place for notifying the primary care physician when his patient has been admitted. The department also should have the names of your admitting physician if you use a hospitalist and respect your choice of admitting team. In my opinion, it is preferable to use one hospital group, so that you get to know your hospitalist team. Once you develop a relationship or "put a face to the name," communication is much easier.

Your hospitalist should also notify you that your patient is admitted. In a study of physician preferences, most preferred to be notified by telephone, although I find that a text message can be direct and succinct. Waiting for a dictated H&P to be faxed is not a good plan, as it may take several days before that information arrives. That's a loss of valuable time to communicate potentially vital patient care information. I also try to educate my patients and their family members to call me at the office if they are admitted to the hospital.

Once you know that your patient is admitted, you may wish to fax your most recent office note, labs, imaging reports, names of specialists, etc. to your hospitalist. This will help her get the big picture of your patient's situation. And it avoids repeating tests and keeps referrals within the same physician group for continuity of care. If I send a patient from my office to the hospital, I give him a copy of this information to hand to the hospital physician.

HOSPITAL DISCHARGES

Although it has always been important to follow-up with your patients upon discharge from the hospital, there are financial incentives to make this happen within *two* business days. Why? Because new Medicare "transitional care" codes now reimburse physicians for the work that we do, such as facilitating home health or therapy referrals, clarifying medications, reviewing records, as long as we follow very specific requirements, including a 2-day communication rule (see Transitional Care Protocols).

If we don't find out that the patient was discharged until *three* days later – you will still do the transitional care work, but 'sayonara' to that additional reimbursement. That makes it all the more important to emphasize to your hospitalist team that you *must be notified* immediately upon the patient's discharge. Again, a phone call, text message or email may be preferable to waiting for a faxed report.

HOSPITAL RECORDS

As Dr. Shandor told us earlier: "Medical records are God." However, it is typical that discharge summaries may not be ready when you see your patient in the office, as the hospital team may not have completed dictations. In fact, studies have shown that discharge summaries average a delay of three weeks in some facilities. [97]

I usually have the patient sign a medical release form at the follow-up appointment after their hospital stay and schedule *another* visit within a week or so to ensure that I understand all relevant issues and can communicate the treatment plan with the patient.

ELEMENTS OF THE ROCK STAR HOSPITAL DISCHARGE SUMMARY

- Discharge medications (and reasons for changes)

- Discharge diagnoses

- Results of procedures or abnormal labs

- Needed appointments or other follow-up

- Pending tests

- Specialist consults and conclusions

TRANSITIONAL CARE PROTOCOL

Disclaimer – Ah, Medicare. They pay the bills, so they make the rules. That being said, the intricacies of documentation and coding are ever changing; therefore always check the most recent updates from CMS before coding any services.[98]

The good news is that Medicare has decided to start reimbursing the work that we have long done for our recently hospitalized patients. The challenge is that we have to follow specific requirements to receive that reimbursement.

As described above, the first requirement for the Transitional Care visit is a patient contact within 2-business days of hospital discharge. The physician or a member of her medical team may do this. The contact may be done by telephone, email, or face-to-face.

Secondly, a face-to-face visit must occur within either 7- or 14- days after discharge, depending on medical complexity:

- CPT Code 99495 – Transitional care management services with moderate medical decision complexity (face-to-face visit within 14 days of discharge);

- CPT Code 99496 – Transitional care management services with high medical decision complexity (face-to-face visit within 7 days of discharge)[99]

To make matters more fun, the billing code must be submitted *on the 30th day* after hospital discharge. No, not 29th, or 31st, but 30th. For more explanation on billing and coding, see the CMS Transitional Care Management Fact Sheet.

TRANSITIONAL CARE TRACKING FORM

Create a Transitional Care tracking form to ensure compliance with Medicare and proper reimbursement. We keep a binder that we check daily to ensure that we are on schedule. Of course, everything goes back to being notified that your patient has been hospitalized!

PATIENT NAME/ ID	DATE OF DISCHARGE	DATE OF CONTACT	DATE OF OFFICE VISIT	BILLING DATE
Mary X. Smith	2/5/2015	2/6/2015 - phone	2/12/2015	3/5/2015
John Z. Doe	3/1/2015	3/2/15 – left voice mail 3/3/15 – left message with wife	Scheduled for 3/8/15	(4/1/15)
Jack Jones	5/2/2015	5/4/15 – no answer at home or cell number		(6/2/15)
Jane Rogers	PENDING			

PREPARING FOR EMERGENCIES

Speaking of hospitalizations, a word about office emergencies. Emergencies will occur, so it is critical to have protocols set up for possible scenarios and to practice with your staff. I have created emergency protocol sheets for the front desk and nursing staff, delineating specific tasks to be done to manage the emergency and to prepare to transition the patient via EMS to the emergency department (Form 6).

EMERGENCY MEDICATIONS

Having the right meds in your cabinets are essential to the Rock Star physician. Your emergency kit (or crash cart, if you have one), needs to contain everything you can think of for a possible office emergency. Epinephrine, in the form of an epi-pen perhaps, Glucagon to reverse hypoglycemia, chewable aspirin, sublingual nitroglycerin, and Benadryl are a good start. You also will want at least two nebulizer machines (during cold season) with albuterol and ipratropium for your wheezers, as well as several oxygen tanks.

For patient comfort, Tylenol or Motrin in the form of tablets or liquid is nice to have on-hand. I also keep liquid prednisone for kids with asthma to get the first dose on-board in the office. Oral steroids have also been shown to decrease the pain of strep throat[100] – I often give one dose in the office. The makings for a GI "cocktail" are useful – a slurry of viscous lidocaine (adults only, please), Maalox or Mylanta, and Donnatal elixir can settle down many upset stomachs.

Other helpful medications to have available are injectable anti-inflammatories like ketorolac (Toradol), a steroid like solumedrol, injectable antiemetics like promethazine, and injectable antibiotics like ceftriaxone (Rocephin). These can sometimes keep your patients out of the emergency department and hospital.

SAMPLE EMERGENCY PROTOCOL FORM

Phone calls:

Caller with acute chest pain, acute shortness of breath, fainting, stroke symptoms ....advise patient to call 911

- when in doubt, ask Dr. Rock Star or err on the side of caution/ 911

Walk-ins:

Notify Dr. Rock Star immediately for:

- acute chest pain
- difficulty breathing, shortness of breath
- severe pain
- stroke symptoms (inability to speak, weakness, numbness)

911 protocol

Dr. Rock Star advises 911 call →

Front desk tasks:

- Place 911 call
- Print out patient demographic sheet
- Make copy of EKG and any pertinent data requested by doctor or EMS team
- Send delegate to meet EMS team downstairs and escort them up
- Notify patient's family member/ friend if so requested

Nursing tasks:

- Obtain EKG if pt is having chest pain
- Get complete vital signs including O2 sat and pain scale
- Bring O2 and tubing
- Bring nebulizer and meds if wheezing
- Bring aspirin, nitroglycerin into room

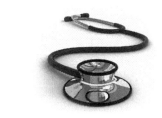

CHAPTER FORTY-FOUR

ROCK STAR CHARTING

As we see from our previous discussion of Transitional Care, physicians spend an immense amount of time tracking patients and documenting care. The medical "chart" is probably one of the most despised elements of the modern medical practice. I say charting rather than documentation, because as doctors, we understand and embrace the idea of creating a written record; the SOAP note (Subjective, Objective, Assessment and Plan), as most of us were originally taught in medical school, for example provides great value for patient care.

Charting, on the other hand, is an entirely different entity. A necessary evil to participate in insurance and government programs, charting has become an unfortunate barrage of checklists and "attestations" to comply with constantly growing regulatory demands. Adding the element of the Electronic Health Record (EHR) with its series of screen changes and multiple "box-clicks" adds a significant amount of time spent on data entry that is often clinically irrelevant, and detracts from direct patient care. In fact, the American Journal of Emergency Medicine showed that emergency room physicians spent "significantly" more time on data entry than on direct patient care.[101]

As government mandates (which were once "incentives") continue to add requirements to show "meaningful use (MU)" of the EHR, the system becomes more burdensome, requiring doctors to either spend more time with the computer on data entry, or hire staff to "fill in the boxes." Not surprisingly, doctors end up spending more time looking at the EHR than they do looking at their patients, which leads to less meaningful patient interaction[102] and more time on what I call "meaning-*less* use."

The Rock Star doctor has to come up with a form of charting that optimizes patient care and minimizes computer time, while utilizing the resources available. This can be a particular challenge with more burdensome EHR systems, more complex patients, and less staff to assist.

Carlos Portu, MD, focuses on ignoring the EHR when he is in the room with the patient. "I have my staff print a copy of the last office note before the visit. When I walk into the exam room I put my paper and pen down, sit down, look straight at the patient and just talk to them. I don't even log into the computer."

While acknowledging that patient charting is a "fine balance," Dr. Portu finds it more patient-focused to minimize computer use in the presence of the patient. "I'll occasionally multi-task a little and order some medications or lab orders, but I try not to dictate or complete my note while I'm in the room with the patient." To follow-up on previous information, his staff prepares for the visit ahead of time, and provides him with copies of recent labs, imaging, or consultant notes in printed form.

To document the current office visit, Dr. Portu takes notes "in my own shorthand" on paper, which he brings back to his office to dictate before seeing his next patient.

Easton Jackson, MD Family Physician from West Valley City, Utah agrees. "If I have an updated problem list, accurate med and allergy list, and a reminder system or tickler file for surveillance labs and studies and preventive services, that's all I need. I don't need the detail of their diabetes follow-up visit in November, 1996."

Other physicians use the computer more interactively during the office visit. One way to engage the patient is to swing the computer monitor to face the patient while you are reviewing information. David Voran, MD, says "Engage the patient by enlisting their help in documenting their visit. Make sure they agree to everything that you're putting in the chart. Start every visit by sitting down with the patient and updating the problem list - make sure they are at your shoulder and watching what you're doing."

While most physicians agree that electronic charting is more a hindrance than a help, there are strategies to make documentation a bit easier.

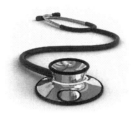

CHAPTER FORTY-FIVE

ROCK STAR CHARTING SECRETS – EFFICIENT NOTE-WRITING TECHNIQUES

COPY-AND-PASTE

While concern about "cloned" notes is rising, it can be extremely effective to use a copy-and-paste form of charting, especially for follow-up visits of multiple chronic medical conditions.

Cloned notes, or notes that are identical to the last visit, and the visit before, and the visit before… are not only fraudulent, but also unfair to yourself and your colleagues. No one wants to waste time flipping through pages of uselessly repeated information. However, the copy and pasted note, when appropriately edited, can be a life-saver in ensuring adequate management of complex medical care and tracking multiple "to-do's," and an element of charting that I use in my practice on a daily basis.

Dr. Roberta Chung does most of her charting by typing and uses the copy-and-paste technique. "I create a detailed assessment and plan for my complex medical patients, which I carry over from the last visit into the current encounter. I then type over and edit the information to make it accurate for the current visit. That way nothing falls off, I can track my preventive care and give myself a reminder each and every time."

Dr. Ariel Cole, a Family Physician who specializes in geriatrics agrees. "Using the last note as a guide is critical in following-up on the many medical issues that seniors have."

USING TEMPLATES AND "QUICK-TEXTS"

Many EHRs have templates or generic data-entry sections for various medical problems – either pre-made or customizable. The benefit to using templates is that they minimize typing/dictating. And they can "count" bullets for coding. The downside is that they are sometimes quite generic and don't always paint the full picture of the patient's issues. Templates tend to be the most useful when the individual physician can personalize them.

"I love to build templates, especially for chronic conditions," says Dr. Portu. He also likes to create quick-texts or phrases that populate when you dictate or type a few characters, as a significant time saver.

Doug Meuser, MD, likes to use templates as well. "It's important to organize your brain to do things repetitively, so you don't miss something important." He creates templates based on evidence-based guidelines, like the European Heart Society and the Joint National Committee for Hypertension (JNC-8). "If it's reproducible, don't type it in every time. Just make sure it's there. Use your EHR to be prompted to do the right things every time."

Another advantage to using templates is that some EHRs can pull the data points from the templates into reports. "Entering data into a good EMR can be really helpful – you can run reports, create flow sheets, and show lab trends. It can give you a 'quick picture' of the patient - there is a lot of good information there," says Jennifer Keehbauch, MD.

USING MEDICAL SCRIBES

Some physicians have begun to incorporate medical scribes into the office environment, something that emergency room physicians have been doing for years. Medical scribes enter data into the medical record, usually in electronic form, as the physician takes the history and performs the physical exam. Scribes are paid $10-20 per hour, and many advocates claim that the return on investment is many-fold, increasing the physician's ability to see more patients as less time is needed for documentation.[103] Using a scribe can be particularly useful for technologically challenged physicians or for those who struggle with keyboard use.

Dr. John Gross, a Family Physician and medical director of St. Anthony's Primary Care, a qualified Patient Center Medical Home, has been using medical scribes for the last few years with good success. "I'm getting my notes done by the end of the day, rather than having them pile up."

In experimenting with medical scribes, I personally found documentation to be much quicker and easier. I had a Medical Assistant in the room with me, clicking the computer as I took the medical history and dictated the physical findings. I kept a separate laptop computer with me so that I could review data while the MA used the desktop computer for charting. Interestingly, I can't do this with my current EHR, because it doesn't allow two users to look at the patient's chart simultaneously!

The challenges that I faced when using a scribe included buy-in from the staff, who felt somewhat overworked by the additional responsibility. Hiring a separate scribe just for that purpose would probably be beneficial, although that person would require a significant amount of training. I found that patients were quite accepting of my use of a scribe - I had little negative feedback from patients for having an additional person in the exam room with us.

DICTATION AND TRANSCRIPTION

Many physicians use dictation for note taking. Traditional dictation to a recording device, typed by a transcriptionist, is beloved by many physicians for accuracy, but can be expensive. Computerized dictation programs, most commonly Dragon Dictation,™ can be effective but demands aggressive training by the physician.

"Just like anything, the more time you put into it at the beginning in terms of setting up your templates and making it learn all the medications you commonly use, that will save you a lot of time later," says Dr. Portu. "If you don't do it at the beginning when you are getting started, inevitably that will cost you ten times as much work later."

Dr. Emily Nabors is one of those fortunate few to still use transcription services in her office. "I complete my dictations after each encounter," she says. "That's when I know the most about the patient. If I come back later, I've forgotten things, and it takes so much longer. It's just the most efficient way – no matter how far behind I am, I finish my dictations. It's hard, but at the end of the day I'm done, and I can walk out the door."

I struggle with completing my notes after each patient encounter, as I get anxious about running further behind, but I have to agree that Dr. Nabors is 100% right. When I force myself to finish my notes in "real time," I manage to finish my day with the majority of my charts completed, rather than leaving them to be finished in the evening or playing catch-up for the rest of the week and into the weekend.

DRAGON DICTATION™ "SECRETS"

It is essential to have the right equipment for dictation programs. A very good microphone, while expensive, is mandatory in getting good voice recognition. Doug Meuser, MD, uses a professional microphone with a boom that allows him to position it perfectly and that keeps him hands-free without having to use an uncomfortable headset. "Everyone made fun of me at first, but now I notice that most of the doctors are using the same thing now."

"Training" the dictation system has to be done regularly, and I have found that running the accuracy optimizer function every week or so seems to improve my results. I have also learned that Dragon does not respond well to yelling.

Dragon can be very useful for creating templates of commonly used phrases, such as a generic treatment plan for viral infections ("URI, likely viral. Rest, fluids, over-the-counter medications reviewed with patient."). I have hundreds. However, once you have trained the system, back up your work! I can't imagine anything more upsetting than losing hours and hours of work because of a system crash.

Be aware of stupid errors in transcription – Dragon often changes "he" to "she" or "will" to "we'll," no matter how many times I train it. It loves to use "C." instead of "see" and never knows when to use "due" or "do." These sort of grammatical errors can make an OCD-type doctor absolutely cuckoo. Consider a disclaimer – I created a Dragon template that I nicknamed "Bad Computer:" "This note was generated using XX EHR, and dictated in part by XX dictation program. Despite the best effort of the dictating physician, there may be grammatical or syntax errors."

DOCUMENTATION - THE BOTTOM LINE: JUST GET 'EM DONE

Ultimately, documentation is critical for successful patient care. The quicker that you finish your notes, the happier you will be – trust me. Procrastinating only makes charting more painful, so try your best to finish your notes in "real time."

ROCK STAR TIP:
Finish your notes in real time as much as possible

Rock Star physician considers *who* will be reviewing and benefiting from the patient record when formulating an office note.

1. **Yourself.** Documentation reminds you of what you were thinking when you saw the patient and describes your differential diagnosis. The note helps you to create a follow up plan – "if this, then that" – and to create a to-do list. It also serves as a guide for your staff – when in doubt, "check the note."

2. **Your staff.** Your staff should be able to use your notes to prepare for the next office visit, to understand the clinical plan, and to answer questions from patients during phone calls. If your staff is trained to check your last note rather than come to you with questions, you will have more time available for your current patient.

3. **Your colleagues.** Covering physicians will appreciate a well-written note that describes the treatment plan and prevents unnecessary repetition of work. A good note allows specialists to

understand the scenario and reason for consultation. Naturally you will never criticize another physician in your documentation!

4. **Your payer.** The notes justify medical necessity and therefore payment. Unfortunately, most reviewers, not physicians themselves, are not looking at your medical differential diagnosis and plan, but rather are counting the "bullets," or elements included in the note (see Billing and Coding Tips). Of course, as Dr. Doug Meuser says: "Say what you do, but do what you say in the medical record. Fraud is bad."

5. **Your malpractice carrier.** You know that old adage "If it isn't documented, it wasn't done." Your note is your best resource and protection in the event of a lawsuit. "Risks, benefits, alternatives, and side effects were discussed with the patient." Ad nauseum.

6. **Your patient.** The chart provides communication to the patient's other physicians and also explains to the patient what transpired during the visit. As Alan Falkoff, MD, a Connecticut Best Family Physician Award Winner says, "Give your patients full access to their medical records. Write your visit notes *for them*. Encourage them to *read* their progress notes. Make it secure for them to access directly into your EMR via a Portal, so no need for printing and wasting paper, ink and printer burnout. That's about as transparent as it gets."

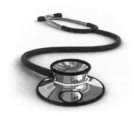

CHAPTER FORTY-SIX

COMPUTER TIPS AND TRICKS –
SURVIVING THE ELECTRONIC RECORD

COMPUTER EQUIPMENT

Use your keyboard effectively. I used to be rather smug about my speedy typing ability, until I realized how little I knew about computer keyboard secrets. Using the "Page Up" and "Page Down" button to speed though pages of notes rather than holding down the stupid mouse. Setting up "hot keys" to open commonly used programs quickly, like your dictation program. Cool keyboard secrets like "Windows + L" to lock your screen, or Ctrl + X to cut, Ctrl + C to copy, and Ctrl + V to paste. I recently learned Ctrl + Z to undo your last action.

Speaking of keyboards, get yourself a good one. Don't use the ancient one that came with your company computer. Pony up for an ergonomic, soft keyed, wireless board – your fingers will thank you. Don't forget to get a wireless optical mouse too!

Go for the biggest computer monitor you can – even better if you can get two monitors side-by-side. When I had a very slow electronic medical record that would take 20-30 seconds to "generate" the office note, I would open the program on both screens, and run them simultaneously. That way I could be working on one chart while another note was generating. Or, I could be checking email or looking up information on the Internet on the other screen.

OFFICE ERGONOMICS

Ergonomics are so important, especially when you are chained to a computer all day long. Unfortunately, IT departments don't often prioritize ergonomics, so you'll probably have to do it yourself. Go on-line and find a nice picture of what your body is supposed to look like while you are sitting at your computer. Try to make yourself look like the little man in the picture – knees at a 90 degree angle, which may require you to prop your feet up on a foot rest; shoulders relaxed, elbows at 90 degrees, wrists slightly flexed, - you'll need your keyboard on a pull-out tray. Your gaze should be towards the top of the monitor screen – my monitor is propped up on "Harrison's Internal Medicine." I knew it would be good for something after medical school. Don't forget good lumbar support (I use a MacKenzie lumbar roll I bought on amazon. com). And try to have armrests on your chair, preferably padded to avoid mouse-induced ulnar neuropathy.

OFFICE LIGHTING

Those fluorescent overhead lights in your office are good for inducing migraines, but not so great for paperwork. Buy a few table or floor lamps, preferably with natural light-type bulbs. Try to angle them to minimize glare on your computer screen.

MENTAL HEALTH IN THE AGE OF THE ELECTRONIC MEDICAL RECORD

- **TRY not to be a perfectionist with your charting.** Accept that with some electronic systems, your notes will look like a third-grader wrote them, with various fonts and text sizes within the note, irregular spacing, and nonsensical elements of meaningful use cluttering up your *truly* useful information. Trying to "fix" the note to look professional is generally an exercise in futility. Repeat the mantra: "My value as a physician is not determined by my electronic medical record notes."

- **ALWAYS BE THINKING about how to outsmart the system.** When pharmacies kept calling me because my electronic system kept defaulting to an expensive brand-name medication, I saved a disclaimer to my medication favorite list: "Computer will default to *Tirosint* – please fill *levothyroxine*." On my prescriptions for doxycycline (which back in the old days I could just write as "doxycycline"), I type "may use either doxycycline monohydrate *or* doxycycline hyclate as available." Or when in doubt of formulary coverage, I write "Proventil HFA inhaler, or may substitute alternate albuterol HFA per patient's insurance formulary."

- **Use disclaimers.** It might not make any difference, but it makes me feel a little better. At the bottom of my notes, I insert a little quick-text that I call "*bad computer*" when I dictate: "This note has been created using the XX Electronic Health Record, and dictated in part by XX Dictation System. Despite the documenting physician's best efforts, there may be errors in grammar or syntax."

- **Look for the positives**. Yes, there are a few. Electronic prescribing can make medication refills quicker and easier; allergy checks can prevent errors (as long as we don't succumb to alarm fatigue), and hey, someone can actually read your writing.

So, here we are, constantly troubleshooting our inadequate computer systems and problem-solving the vast daily minutiae that make up our health care system. The amount of work and mental energy that we expend almost becomes second nature – we often don't even realize how above and beyond we go in caring for our patients. Sometimes we even martyr ourselves on an altar of paperwork, coming in before the staff in the morning, leaving late at night, working on charts on vacation… sound familiar? In order to become a Rock Star physician, we have to empower ourselves and our profession, and avoid selling ourselves short.

ROCK STAR RULE #11:

Don't sell yourself short

Remember those 20,000 hours of training that primary care physicians get? We are highly skilled so we should be working up to the level of our training and coding maximally for reimbursement. For example, why send your patient to a dermatologist when you can do a simple biopsy? Why refer them to an orthopedist for a joint injection? These procedures also make for a lovely break from all the cognitive work that we do all day dealing with chronic disease management.

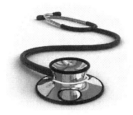

CHAPTER FORTY-SEVEN

OFFICE PROCEDURES AND WOUND CARE

Why *wouldn't* a physician want to do office procedures? With proper training and the right tools, procedures are great for patient care, well reimbursed, and well, just plain fun.

Think about it. You can remove a skin lesion or do a knee injection in less time *and* with better reimbursement than any regular E/M office visit. And most importantly, your patient is happy because she didn't have to take the time and expense to see a specialist.

The Rock Star physician is ready and able to perform common procedures such as skin biopsies (shave, punch, and excisional), ingrown toenail removal, joint drainage and injections, incision and drainage of abscesses, cysts, and paronychia, and minor laceration repairs. Even more simple procedures include snipping off skin tags with an iris scissor, cauterizing an umbilical granuloma or treating a wart with liquid nitrogen spray.

For some doctors, doing in-office aesthetic procedures along with a conventional medical practice can be a nice break from the more esoteric aspects of medicine and financially fulfilling with the right patient population. Personally, I choose not to offer aesthetic services – as a believer in the Golden Rule, I personally would rather see a Board Certified Facial Plastic Surgeon than an FP like myself. But to each his own.

The key to success is having an established protocol for each procedure that you perform in the office.

1. MAKE SURE THAT YOU ARE PROFICIENT IN THE PROCEDURE.

If you didn't have the opportunity to practice many procedures in your residency, there are many courses at continuing medical education conferences. For example, I learned how to perform a shoulder injection at a Family Medicine conference – after an instructional lecture we had the opportunity to practice on mannequins under the tutelage of an orthopedic specialist. Another way to gain expertise is to find a physician mentor that does procedures in the office. As they taught us in med school: "See one, do one, teach one."

And if it has been awhile since you performed a given procedure, take a few minutes to review the anatomy and proper technique in the medical literature before you begin.

Be sure to know your limitations – when in doubt, refer the patient to the appropriate specialist.

2. OBTAIN INFORMED CONSENT.

Keep a standard informed consent form in your exam rooms or print one from your EHR if that is possible. Since these are relatively minor procedures, you don't expect something to go wrong, but it's always the right thing to let the patient know of the potential risks or side effects.

3. CREATE A PROTOCOL FOR EVERY PROCEDURE.

Take the time to breakdown each procedure into individual steps and create an organized list of supplies and actions required. Using this protocol, any medical assistant should be able to quickly ready the exam room for the procedure. Include a plan for follow-up and a patient handout if necessary for after the procedure. Dr. Douglas Meuser still uses protocols that he created during his residency days. "I keep an index card for each procedure that I do – it's a script that I follow."

4. HAVE THE RIGHT TOOLS.

Having the proper equipment for a procedure makes all the difference. When I worked in an underserved county clinic, we often had to make-do with adaptations. No nail elevator for ingrown toenail removal? Use the flat of an iris scissor. No finger splints? Try a tongue depressor and plenty of paper tape. That being said, having the correct instruments makes a procedure so much simpler and a lot more fun.

For example, having the right sized hemostat makes suturing go from absolute hell (as the needle slips out of your grasp over and over again) to a piece of cake. Ever tried removing a foreign body from a vagina without a long-handled ring forceps? Good luck. The right tools really do make the difference.

Make sure that your patients know that you offer office procedures! Several of my patients have reported going to Urgent Care centers or specialists for procedures that could have easily been cared for in the practice.

WOUND CARE

I love wound care. Why send your patient to a wound clinic when you can take care of most wounds in your office?

If you didn't get much experience in wound care during your training, again, plenty of courses are available or your local wound care center may be happy to have you spend some time shadowing their medical team. Again, half the battle is having the right equipment and supplies at hand.

1. CLEANSING

Good news. You don't really need anything fancy to clean most wounds. Just use good old soap and water, and plenty of it. In fact, using iodine or hydrogen peroxide is not even recommended for open wounds.

Get out *all* foreign material, especially in cases of "road rash." I'll never forget a patient who came in with a bulging, fluctuant, and infected knot on her forehead at a sutured laceration site. Upon draining the lesion, several hunks of gravel came out! Not good.

2. DEBRIDEMENT

As above, removing foreign material, dead skin, blood clots, pus, etc is essential to good wound healing. I like to say that necrotic skin is *not* nature's Band-Aid.

To minimize pain, we keep topical lidocaine in the form of EMLA cream and apply it to more painful wounds with an occlusive dressing for 30 minutes to an hour before attempting debridement. Injectable lidocaine is also an option for deeper wounds that require exploration and debridement.

3. USE "GOO"

Why use topical antibiotic ointments when good old-fashioned goo of any kind will do? A dab of Vaseline, or surgi-lube will keep a wound moist, and eliminate the chance of allergic reactions to topical antibiotics.

4. KEEP IT COVERED

Every office needs a hefty supply of gauze and paper tape. Non-stick pads can be helpful (although using goo may be adequate to keep the gauze from sticking), and having tube gauze is a pure delight. Tube gauze comes in a variety of widths, and can be cut to size and placed over an extremity to keep dressings intact without using tape. It's beautiful, especially for adhesive-allergic patients.

Other helpful bandaging techniques include the use of IV-site dressings, which form a nice, waterproof occlusive wrap and a variety of alginate dressings for difficult wounds like sacral ulcers.

5. USE COMPRESSION

I *love* compression wraps for swelling or venous stasis wounds on the lower extremities. Compression can be a hard sell for some patients, but it can make all the difference in speeding the healing process.

Chronic weeping wounds such as lymphedema or venous stasis wounds often respond well to Unna wraps, a medicated moist form of compression dressings. A snug, but not over-tight compression wrap, sock or stocking has been shown to improve healing time in vascular wounds. If you can't convince your patient to wear a medical grade stocking, a pair of "Miracle Socks," available at many retailers may be helpful.

As with all medical treatment, make sure that you review the guidelines for the indications and use of compression in wound care.

6. TAKE OPPORTUNITY TO UPDATE TETANUS VACCINES

At this time, Medicare doesn't cover routine preventive tetanus vaccines. However, they *do* cover vaccines (tetanus-toxoid) for tetanus-prone wounds if the last vaccine was more than 10 years prior. This is a golden opportunity to get your patient vaccinated.

7. FREQUENT FOLLOW-UP

Reassess the wound within 1-2 days of the initial visit. Remove all wrapping, cleanse the wound, perform additional debridement if necessary, and reapply the appropriate dressing. Repeat this process every few days until the wound is fully healed. Slow or poorly healing wounds should, of course, be referred to a wound specialist.

8. KNOW YOUR LIMITATIONS

As always, an atypical or non-healing wound warrants referral to a dermatologist or wound care specialist. Any evidence of vascular or neurologic compromise necessitates an immediate surgical consultation.

ROCK STAR RULE #11, EXPANDED:
Don't sell yourself short by undercoding

One of the main reasons that we spend so much time on our charting is so that we can get paid. The Rock Star doctor uses the medical record to optimally capture charges and accurately code for reimbursement. This will also avoid the common problem of undercoding that represents a significant loss of revenue for many office practices.

– DISCLAIMER: Although a Rock Star physician, I am not claiming to be an expert on coding and billing. Rules are constantly changing. So, it's critical to review the most current coding guidelines and to have your billing audited regularly by a professional. All documentation should include only those elements that are reasonable and medically necessary for the clinical problems being evaluated.

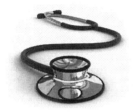

CHAPTER FORTY-EIGHT

BILLING AND CODING TIPS FOR ROCK STAR OFFICE VISITS

In residency, when did you learn how to organize your own medical office, to design a schedule or how to correctly bill? My program offered a Practice Management course, a week or two long. I remember our faculty member saying, "Don't worry about these E/M (evaluation and management) codes; a new version is about to come out and will change everything." That was in 2002. Fast-forward to 2015, and these "future changes" are still being predicted.

Needless to say, medical coding is complicated. In fact, it is estimated that Family Physicians undercode about 30% of the time. Over time, this can add up to a significant amount of lost revenue.

The main problem is that doctors tend to sell themselves short, underestimating their medical decision-making (MDM), which is the key to medical coding and billing.

Volumes (literally – the latest American Medical Association Current Procedural Terminology - or CPT - coding book is 600 pages long) exist to help explain the nuances of medical coding. For the Rock Star physician, we will focus on the elements needed to code a 99214, one of the most common level of services in primary care for an established patient. And, it's one that often goes undercoded.

To code a 99214, you must have two out of three of the following medical decision making (MDM) elements: Problems, Data, and Risk.[104] [105]

PROBLEMS:

A "problem" is anything that you as a physician are addressing. It is separated into "points" depending on the complexity of the problem. To have enough problems for a 99214, you need "3" points. Obviously a more complex problem earns more points.

A *new* problem requiring work-up is 4 points, while a new problem without the need for more work-up is 3 points.

- Examples: *New* diagnosis of diabetes will need lab tests, etc. 4 points. New problem of back pain, but no additional testing needed. 3 points.

Bottom line: if you address any *new* problem in an office visit, you have earned one out of the three elements of 99214 MDM.

Established problems earn fewer points, but can be added together. An established problem, getting worse = 2 points.

- Examples: known diabetes, with Hgb A1c worsening. Or high blood pressure uncontrolled.

An established problem that is stable or better = 1 point. You can have as many established problems as you can handle in an office visit.

- Examples: Diabetes, controlled. HTN, controlled. Hyperlipidemia, controlled. Ooh, look, you got 3 points, and now qualify for a 99214 by problem points!

An established problem, getting worse (2) WITH a stable established problem (1) earns a total of 3 points. So, count the problems, add up the points, and if you get at least 3 points, you are looking at a potential 99214.

DATA:

"Data" are anything that you use to make your medical decisions. You need "3" data points for a 99214. Essentially, you get one point for each of the following: review/order labs, review/order radiology, review/order tests like EKG, echo, PFTs. You get 2 points for reviewing/ summarizing old records. It is not that common to get 3 data points in a typical office visit – but if you meet the criteria for problems and risk, data points don't matter anyway (remember, you only need 2/3).

RISK:

To qualify for a 99214, you need to have at least moderate risk. For most of us in primary care, the bottom line is that any *prescription drug management* = *moderate risk*. In other words, if you're writing a prescription, stopping a medication or changing a medication, you are now at moderate risk.

To earn a 99214, you have to have *two* out of the *three* elements of MDM. Most of the time, we end up using Problem + Risk, as Data points seem to be a little tougher to earn.

For example, a patient presenting with back pain (new problem = 3 points) is prescribed a prescription pain medication (Moderate Risk) = 99214.

Or take a classic primary care patient with hypertension, controlled, and uncontrolled diabetes, for whom you are adjusting medication = 99214. Boom.

I know that it's hard to believe. You are a Rock Star, after all, and medical conditions like these might be something you could manage in your sleep. Doesn't matter. You earned that 99214 fair and square. *Don't sell yourself short.*

Oh, but don't forget to ensure that your history and/or physical exam match up with your MDM. It's really not hard for the average primary care patient. Here's the bare minimum.

HISTORY OF PRESENT ILLNESS (HPI)

The HPI requires 4 elements OR documenting the status of 3 chronic problems.

Elements of history may involve description of symptoms, duration, exacerbating and relieving factors, location, and concurrent symptoms.

Examples:

HPI 4 elements for patient with a "cough:" cough x 3 days (1), productive of white phlegm (2), getting worse (3), Nyquil helps for a few hours (4).

Status of 3 chronic problems: Diabetes, controlled with medication, no hypoglycemia (1). HTN, elevated, forgot to take meds for the last few days (2). Hyperlipidemia – tolerating statin without side effects (3).

REVIEW OF SYSTEMS (ROS)

Next, you only need *two* elements of the ROS. That's right, I said two.

Example:

ROS: No chest pain or shortness of breath. No fever or weight loss.

PAST HISTORIES

Finally, you need to note that you have reviewed and/or updated at least *one* historical element (medical, surgical, family or social history).

Example: Pt is a nonsmoker. Or: PMH reviewed.

See how easy!

THE 99214 PHYSICAL EXAMINATION

You need 12 "bullets," or details, from the physical exam to earn a 99214. I won't go into detail here, only because you probably won't need the exam elements, since 99% of the time you can easily qualify for a 99214 with your history + MDM. Also, see "The extremely-directed physical exam" section.

PHYSICAL EXAM - COUNTING BULLETS

For a "detailed" physical examination, there must be documentation of 2 bullets from 6 organ systems. A "comprehensive" physical examination requires 2 bullets from 9 different organ systems.

By my count, at least 4 organ systems can be examined "just by looking" and another 3 by brief touch: Constitutional (three vital signs, general appearance), Eyes (inspection of conjunctiva and lids, examination of pupils/ irises), EENT (external appearance of ears and nose, assessment of hearing), Neck (trachea, symmetry, thyroid), Musculoskeletal (gait and station, inspection of digits and nails, inspection of muscular areas),

Psychiatric (judgment, insight, orientation, mood), Skin (inspection, palpation). Listen to the heart and lungs and you've got another 2 organ systems. Take your pick of any of the remainder organ systems for your 9th and final system – check the neck, palpate the abdomen, check lymph nodes.

THE "99215"

Let's also look at a high complexity situation, or 99215. Again, it's not as difficult as one might imagine.

1. *New* problem requiring additional evaluation or established problem with severe flare or side effect from medication

2. Life or body function threatening situation, mental status change

My rule of thumb: if I call 911 or send someone to the emergency room, automatic 99215. If I am really worried about someone, it's probably going to be a 99215. If I'm really scared that the medicine I am prescribing will have serious side effects and I've got to monitor the patient ultra-closely, 99215.

Interestingly, the decision not to resuscitate or to de-escalate care because of poor prognosis, as in a hospice patient, is considered a high-risk situation and qualifies for a 99215.

The history elements are slightly more demanding than the 99214, with the main differences being that the 99215 requires a *complete* review of systems (10 systems), and a complete past history review (medical, family, *and* social).

A CAVEAT ON THE "99204"

Don't mistake the ease of a 99214 with a 99204. The latter is the code for a *new* patient visit, and the elements are more complex, requiring 3/3 elements rather than 2/3. In particular, history and physical examinations must be comprehensive, including a complete ROS and PE.

I'm a big fan of the E/M University (www.emuniversity.com) to learn more details about medical coding, with many examples and practice exercises. Also, I strongly recommend that you make yourself a chart to review when you are learning the ropes - don't just "gestalt it" unless you are a pro!

AND DON'T FORGET THE "99211" AND "99212"

You are a doctor. Therefore, *you* should never be coding a 99211. This is a nursing code for evaluation ordered by the physician, classically a blood pressure check. Don't let me catch you coding a 99211. Your nurse, on the other hand, should certainly be reporting a 99211 when indicated.

On the other hand, a 99212 should be used liberally. If you looked at the patient and talked to the patient about *anything* medical, you should be coding a 99212 at a minimum.

Example: Patient comes in for a wound check and dressing change. The nurse has the wound unwrapped, you take a look, order the dressings, and plan the follow-up. 99212. Or a patient's husband asks you to take a look in his ear during his wife's visit. 99212.

I know, it sounds too easy. Billing just for a quick ear check? That's because as physicians we *sell ourselves short!* When I called the plumber for a stopped up drain, he opened it up, pulled out a wad of hair (I know, I know, gross), and charged me a hundred bucks. I bet he didn't feel guilty about charging me for something so simple, so why should we?

CODING CHARTS

I recommend making yourself a little chart and posting it on the wall where you do your documentation. If you work in multiple settings, such as an in-patient hospital setting or nursing home, the codes will be even more complex, so charts are especially helpful. I keep multiple charts on my wall to double-check that I am meeting the bullet criteria. Here's an example of basic outpatient office visit charts:

SAMPLE OFFICE VISIT CODING CHEAT SHEET

Established patient – must meet 2/3 criteria (history OR examination)

	99212	99213	99214	99215
History	1-3	1-3	4+	4+
ROS	-	1	2-9	10
Past histories	-	-	1	3 (full)
Exam	1-5	6	12	18
MDM	Straight-forward	LOW	MODERATE	COMPLEX/HIGH RISK

New patient – and don't forget, you have to meet BOTH history and examination criteria, not just two out of three, as required with an established patient!

	99201	99202	99203	99204	99205
History	1-3	1-3	4+	4+	4+
ROS	-	1	2-9	10	10
Past histories	-	-	1	3 (full)	3 (full)
Exam	1-5	6	12	18	18
MDM	Straight-forward	Straight-forward	LOW	MODERATE	COMPLEX/HIGH RISK

Time based documentation

New patient	Established patient
99201 = 10 minutes	99211 = -
99202 = 20 minutes	99212 = 10 minutes
99203 = 30 minutes	99213 = 15 minutes
99204 = 45 minutes	99214 = 25 minutes
99205 = 60 minutes	99215 = 40 minutes

TIME BASED DOCUMENTATION

Time based documentation can really come in handy when you have to spend the bulk of your visit either "counseling or coordinating care." For example, it will likely come into play with the patient who comes in severely depressed or has a stack of forms for you to fill out.

The requirements for this coding are specific. There must be a certain amount of face-to-face time with "greater than 50%" of that time spent on counseling or coordinating care.

While you don't have to do lots of documentation for history or physical, you *do* have to document the time spent, both total and counseling time, and details on the counseling/coordination of care activity.

Example: "This was a 45 minute face-to-face office visit, with greater than 50% (30 minutes) spent counseling on depression symptoms, treatment options, and medication choices including side effects, suicide warning, and arranging referral to psychologist." New patient = 99204. Established patient = 99215.

ROCK STAR RULE #12:

Make your mental health a priority

289

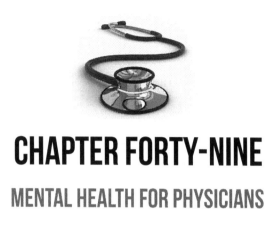

CHAPTER FORTY-NINE

MENTAL HEALTH FOR PHYSICIANS

If the above section hasn't gotten you thinking about mental health, then nothing will! In earlier sections of this book, I've jokingly referred to seeking psychological help for various issues. But in all seriousness, the Rock Star doctor is not afraid to get help dealing with whatever issues are causing stress, whether relatively minor issues like your dread of electronic medical records, more serious problems like compassion fatigue or even personal demons.

The reality is that doctors have the highest rate of suicide of any profession, with male physicians having a 1.4 times higher rate of suicide, and women 2.3 times higher compared with the general population.[106] Studies suggest that this increased rate of suicide is due to undiagnosed and untreated depression, inadequate mental health treatment, and increased problems related to job stress.

I firmly advocate for every doctor to have his own mental health specialist. Guess what? What we do is tough! We have to interact with up to 20-30 individual personalities every single day, while maintaining a sometimes forced friendly and cheerful persona. As Carlos Portu, MD, says, "I have to flip a switch from whatever is going on in my own life and make the patient feel that they are the most important thing going on with me today."

Oh, and meanwhile, we also have to actually provide medical care! And don't forget about the insurance authorizations, medication denials, rejected claims… etc. It's enough to make the most mentally stable person come home and feel like kicking the dog… or husband.

"My wife says I don't have a meaningful conversation with her between Monday and Friday," says Dr. Portu with a laugh. "That's because I've had 30 conversations already today. It's very, very hard to walk into a room and be happy and peppy that many times per day. Unless you've done what we do it's hard to understand what it's like."

Maybe that's why divorce rates among physicians in some studies have been reported to be 10% to 20% higher than those in the general population. In 1997, psychiatrists were found to have the highest rate at around 50%; surgeons next at 33%; and the profession as a whole with a divorce rate of 29%. Women physicians and those who married while still in med school had higher rates of divorce.[107]

Physicians also are not immune to problems with alcohol and substance abuse. While overall rates of impairment are similar between physicians and the general public, rates of prescription drug abuse were five times higher among physicians.[108]

So, other than the obvious, what contributes to our stress level? While much of the stress of being a physician comes from the nature of medical practice, studies have shown certain traits and characteristics typical of the types of people that become doctors, in particular, perfectionism.

One of the most serious causes of distress in physicians is the perception of having made a mistake – a memory that can haunt the physician for years.[109] We are often hesitant to share our concerns with our colleagues. Instead we internalize the pain of making a mistake, which is inevitable at some point in medical practice. Physicians who have made a medical error, whether a serious mistake or a "near-miss," reported anxiety about future errors (61%), loss of confidence (44%), sleeping difficulties (42%), reduced job satisfaction (42%), and harm to their reputations (13%).[110]

Other studies have suggested that errors can increase the physician's risk of depression, substance abuse, suicide, and posttraumatic stress disorder. Self-perceived errors are associated with reduced quality of life, increased burnout, and depression.[111]

"The hardest part about a bad outcome is forgiving yourself. You have to accept that you can't know it all, and bad things will happen even though you did your best," says Roberta Chung, MD.

After a medical error, studies show that doctors need support. Sharing experiences with psychological specialists or trusted colleagues helped 63% of patients to progress past the medical error.[112]

But often we are advised by risk managers and malpractice lawyers *not* to talk about potential errors. What isolation! How can we vent, receive affirmation of competence, get opinions from others?

One way to reach out for support is through physician-only websites, like Sermo. This anonymous website for physicians-only is a resource for sharing feelings and getting feedback from others that may have had similar experiences.

Another major source of emotional stress in physicians comes from "the culture of medical training." We are trained to work long hours without complaint, put aside our own physical health and comfort – in other words, "suck it up." We learn to harden our hearts against the emotions of suffering, fear, mortality, and the limits of medical knowledge. Over time, this form of coping can become "maladaptive," leading to psychological distress.

So, knowing all of this, why do doctors neglect their own psychological care? Well, for many of the same reasons as our patients – the imagined stigma and fear of possible repercussions from medical boards or employers, a sense of failure of 'needing help,' denial, lack of trust in others, procrastination or waiting until hitting rock bottom, and a lack of time.[113] Meanwhile, we are haranguing our patients to do exactly what we need to be doing!

The Rock Star doctor is not embarrassed to admit when he needs a little help getting through a tough time. In fact, he is in an ideal position to use his positive experiences to encourage others in their journey of improved mental health. The more vocal and casual we are about mental health ("sure, doesn't everyone have a psychologist?"), the more we remove the elements of stigma, silence, and secretiveness. Then, we all win.

I am quite vocal about acknowledging my own regular psychology visits. I like to say that I go "every three weeks, whether I need it or not." Because even if today everything is going well, that doesn't mean that tomorrow I won't face a new life stress. I work with my psychologist not only on my own personal issues, but to strategize on how to better care for my patients in dealing with their psychological issues. I often tell my patients: "Since the people who *really* need to see a psychologist won't go, the rest of us have to!"

Although most everyone could probably benefit from a regular psychology appointment, there are plenty of non-clinical ways to improve your own psychological health.

- Exercise

- Self Care

- Nature

- Fun (as Paul Marsolek says, "If you're not having fun, you're not trying hard enough!")

- Spirituality

- Relationships

- Vacation/Leisure

A study found that of various wellness promotion strategies used by physicians, a positive approach to life, focusing on successes, and maintaining a balance in life was found to most increase psychological well-being scores.[114]

One way to improve work-life balance is to consider taking off one weekday every week. I started doing this with a half day, but soon realized that I would end up stretching the day later as I worked in additional patients or found tasks that needed to be done. The day ended up more as a ¾ day than a half! Taking a weekday off allows you to take care of your own needs – like your doctor, dentist, psychiatrist, financial advisor, etc. Somehow I manage to fill that day off with appointments nearly every week – how did I manage beforehand? To maintain your income, you may want to work a 10-hour four-day work week, which may also be beneficial to your patients, who may appreciate early or late hour appointments.

STRESS REDUCTION TECHNIQUES –
SELF-VISUALIZATION AND RELAXATION TECHNIQUES

Volumes have been written about how to meditate, usually advocating 20 minutes once or twice a day. Yeah, right. If I had 20 minutes once or twice a day free, I wouldn't need to meditate.

So instead, let's focus on a few things that we can do in seconds to no more than a few minutes.

1. **Breathing techniques**. Slow, deep breathing has been shown to lower blood pressure, stress levels, improve sleep, and maybe even reduce feelings of pain. It just takes a few seconds and can be done between patients, in the morning, at bedtime, whenever.

2. **Visualization**. This is a great distraction technique to remove recurrent, perseverating negative thoughts: close your eyes, and imagine a train carrying a load of something pleasant (daisies?). The train pushes the negative thought off the track, and you watch the cars go by until the train passes. Open your eyes. The thought pops back in? Repeat the train exercise.

3. **Stretching/yoga**. An entire yoga class would be great, but just a few stretches with deep breathing can reinvigorate you and lower stress.

4. **Guided imagery**. There are lots of books, websites, and programs that teach guided imagery, basically just a deliberate effort to imagine yourself in a certain environment – your "happy place." Close your eyes, and see yourself in that place – including the smells, sounds, feels, etc.

5. **Mindfulness.** Again, tons of courses, books, websites. The idea is to be ultra-aware of your body, your surroundings, your emotions, and how you interact with the world around you in a "non-judgmental" way, if only for a few moments. "I find that

being grateful for what I have really works for me," says Jennifer Keehbauch, MD. "When I find myself stressing, I redirect myself to being grateful."

6. **Positive self-talk**. "I'm good enough, I'm smart enough..." As with visualization above, replace a negative thought with a positive one. It doesn't work to "tell yourself" to stop thinking negatively – kind of like the old "don't think about the pink elephant" game. Instead, you have to deliberately change the negative thought to a positive one. This also goes for envisioning positive results – if you're called into a meeting with the boss, instead of thinking the worst, imagine something positive – probably a well-deserved raise. If not, you can always go to #7:

7. **Venting – in a safe way**. Journaling is a classic example of safely venting. "I can't deal with stressful thoughts during my work day, so I write my concerns down and give myself permission to think about them later," says Dr. Keehbauch, who uses the Note section of her iPhone. "I find that when I take the time to review them later, they aren't as 'potent' – they've lost some of the emotion of the moment." Another way of venting is to use an anonymous physician website like Sermo.com to share your dilemmas, worries, and anger. Likely you will find others that feel the same way, or at least you can get it off your chest.

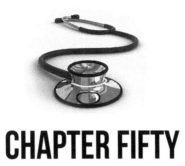

CHAPTER FIFTY

SPECIAL STRESSES FOR WOMEN PHYSICIANS

The good news is that most women physicians seem to "enjoy better than average physical health and lead satisfying and productive lives." On the other hand, some studies report that women have higher than average rates of depression, anxiety, marital problems, and substance abuse, with 49% of women physicians reporting usually having high levels of stress (sounds low to me!). [115]

In addition to the usual causes of physician stress, women also have challenges with high expectations, both from themselves and others, and balancing multiple roles at home and at work.

Dr. Roberta Chung, Family Physician and mother of three young children says, "There is such an expectation of having to be a great mother and wife, as well as a good physician. Something has to give. I can't be everything to everybody. It's hard to find balance."

Women face special stress when it comes to child-rearing and family responsibilities. Dr. Ariel Cole, Family Florida Hospital Geriatric Fellowship Director and mother of two, feels the pressure of balancing roles. "There is definitely a stigma towards part-time work and taking time off from work. I feel like people think less of me for working part-time. 'Why do we waste all our money on women who don't work full-time?' And graduates who elect not to work to stay home full-time with young kids are not looked on favorably at all."

In general, women physicians are more likely to carry the responsibility of caring for families after work hours. Even in physician marriages, wives are more likely to adjust their careers to focus on family than husbands. And while studies show that women and men have equal career motivation, having children has a negative impact on women physician careers, slowing career progression of women in academic medicine.[116]

Children seem to be the common denominator, with childless (or perhaps we should say child-free) physicians working fewer hours than physicians with children.[117] Women physicians also show an improvement in mental health once child rearing is complete, with women physicians over age 50 or with children over age 19 reporting the best mental health.

Women physicians with children at home spend fewer hours on professional activities and more time on childcare than men physicians with children. Combining professional and "unwaged" activities, women with children work more than men with children, putting in an average of 90.5 hours per week, while men averaged 68.6 hours.[118]

Women often choose to focus on child raising during the early years of their career, but often return to full-time work when children are older. Dr. Ariel Cole: "It was very important to me to take my twelve weeks of

FMLA time off with my first child. Although I am working part-time while my children are pre-school age, I fully plan to return to full-time medicine once they are older."

Interestingly, when women do return full-time into the workforce they actually catch up with their male colleagues, with studies showing that academic women physicians publish more scientific studies – increasing and actually exceeding men – in the later stage of their careers. However, women tend to hold fewer leadership positions than men, probably due to a slower start in academic productivity due to child rearing. [119]

Women with children are often subject to "micro-inequalities." For example, while Dr. Cole is paid a reduced salary, she is also penalized for working part-time by not being eligible for additional perks that full-time faculty members receive. "Even though I'm at home, I'm often still working, checking the computer, doing medication refills."

Over the entire length of their careers, women physicians earn less than men physicians, despite increased work productivity – with women seeing substantially more patients per office hour (about 17% more, on average, over time). Women primary care physicians earn about 70% as much as men physicians. [120]

Here's something disheartening for women that wish to become physicians: studies indicate that the average woman would be financially better off becoming a *Physician Assistant* than a physician! When the cost of medical school education and the gender wage gap are factored in, women physicians "simply don't work enough hours to amortize their upfront investment in medical school." [121] What?!

As if that weren't enough, women also experience stress related to discrimination and lack of role models and support. I remember a not-to-be-named male administrator asking me if I had children. When I responded in the negative, he said, "Good, I'll be able to get more work out of you."

Even more upsetting is the fact that 73% of women physicians have reported verbal abuse while at work, with 33% reporting physical assault at work! And while depression rates are about the same as the general public, women physicians have higher rates of successful suicide, with more than half of women physicians experiencing some type of psychiatric illness in their lifetime.[122]

"We put so much pressure on ourselves to be perfect," says Emily Nabors, MD, Family Physician and mother of one. "We tend to take things home more often. We take on patients problems, and I think that we are told more problems by our patients than male physicians, and tend to spend more time with our patients."

Studies indicate that Dr. Nabors is correct. Compared to male physicians, women spend 40-60% more time talking with patients; they also engage in more positive talk, partnership building, question asking, and information giving.[123] Patients speak more to female physicians than to male physicians and disclose more biomedical and psychosocial information. Interestingly, patients are also more assertive toward female physicians and tend to interrupt them more. [124]

Women physicians see more female patients, with four out of every five visits being from women. Women physicians also see more patients with complex psychosocial problems compared with their male colleagues, spend longer with patients, and perform more preventive services than male physicians such as pap tests and mammograms.[125]

However, women physicians have less work control then men regarding day-to-day aspects of the practice like scheduling or volume of patient load. Is it any wonder that women had 1.6 times the odds of reporting burnout compared with men? This burnout significantly increases with working more than 40 hours per week.[126]

So how do we cope with this increased burnout? Since we can't depend on institutional change, we have to find methods of coping with this increased stress. Studies show that the odds of burnout were 40% less when they had the support of colleagues, spouse or significant other for balancing work and home issues. Dr. Emily Nabors advises, "Psychology is a really good idea, particularly when your job becomes overwhelming. I have many physician friends who have found therapy to be very helpful in giving insight and perspective."

Additionally, women need to work to support each other and provide positive role modeling to the next generation of women physicians.

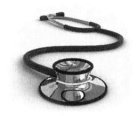

CHAPTER FIFTY-ONE

FINDING WORK-LIFE BALANCE AND SATISFACTION

Wouldn't it be just great if you just loved what you did for a living? I used to get jealous when I heard people raving about their jobs and how lucky they are to get paid for what they enjoy. You know the kind – they're usually an artist, a chef or maybe a cruise ship director.

Well, reality check. Most of us work because we have to, not always because we're necessarily living our dream. Hey, maybe you do, and that's great. But if you don't wake up excited every single day to go into work, you have to find something that you *do* love about your job. And then cling to that thought with a passion.

The good news is that by following the Rock Star rules, you will have the tools to decrease work stress and increase your job satisfaction.

"Work-life balance is different for everyone, and it changes throughout your life. You have to figure out what is important to you, and try to work your career around that," says Roberta Chung, MD. "When you find the right balance you look forward to work and it energizes you – but isn't 'everything' to you. I love going to work now because if fulfills a part of me but isn't the whole of me."

Dr. Chung found this balance by adjusting her schedule from a 10-15 minute visit to a 20-40 minute visit. "Spending more time with patients provides me with a better balance. It helps prevent burnout. My hours didn't change, but now I can practice medicine the way I want to."

"You have to find the 'hat' you like," says Dr. Doug Meuser. "This makes work fun, and prevents burn out." He suggests that doctors consider a transition if they are miserable at their job or look for something to keep their practice interesting. "If you have a financial commitment to your practice, look for things that you can incorporate that interest you – research, procedures; something that you love and can have fun with."

I personally found that when I transitioned from a corporate structure to a small, family-owned practice I was suddenly empowered – and found myself loving my job for the first time in years.

Paul Marsolek, physician advisor, suggests that doctors: "Use what you have, your strengths, purposely." He points to a physician he mentored that struggled with patient satisfaction, which was affecting her compensation. "When we evaluated the data, we found that her reviews from senior citizens were through the roof! So we transformed her practice into a geriatric focus, with instant improvement in her total patient satisfaction and her stress levels."

FOCUS ON PATIENT CARE

Despite the frustrations of being a doctor, most physicians find their careers rewarding – and the majority of physicians report that their favorite part of their job is patient care and forming relationships.[127] "I miss patient care," says Beth Shandor, DO, a board-certified Internal Medicine physician who now works as an administrator. "I went into medicine to help people."

"The best part of being a doctor is that people trust you with their lives," says Dr. Emily Nabors. "You have a relationship that makes you privy to information that others don't know."

Dr. Jennifer Keehbauch, who opened an after-hours clinic for the underserved at her residency program advises, "Find something that ignites the fire in you. I started working with the underserved in college and medical school, and this reminds me of why I went into medicine. It helps to work with grateful people. "

ROCK STAR TIP:

To stay focused on relationships, keep a folder where you can put patient notes, thank you cards or any type of positive feedback that you receive. Pull it out when you are feeling discouraged with medicine

Another way to focus on relationships is to surround yourself with positive people. Have fun with your staff – bring in lunch a few times per month. Celebrate birthdays. Spend time with valued colleagues. "Hang out with other doctors, vent, share ideas," recommends Dr. Jennifer Keehbauch, the President of the Florida Academy of Family Physicians. "Join a local physician group. Find a mentor."

REMEMBER WHY YOU WENT INTO MEDICINE

Aside from relationships, "Being very good at what I do/Finding answers and diagnoses" was listed as the second most rewarding aspect of being a physician on Medscape's 2014 Physician Report. The value of making a diagnosis and changing a person's life for the better can't be underestimated. And remembering these moments can keep you going on the more mundane days. Keeping a list of success stories or cool diagnoses that you've made in your folder can help you focus on the good that you have done.

Dr. Emily Nabors enjoys working with medical students, which reminds her of why she became a doctor. "Teaching medical students increases my satisfaction as a physician. It's nice to see young people and to find out what and how they are learning. I love sharing Family Medicine with them."

I know that I felt joy when a medical student told me that she selected Family Medicine as her career choice because of her experience with me in a rural clinic. And I was so proud when two of my pre-medical student "shadows" were accepted to medical school.

Working with medical students is also a great reminder of how far we've come. "Having students keeps you young and inquisitive," says Jennifer Keehbauch, MD. "I forget every July how 'green' they are, and we were at one point."

And indeed, as I listen to med students talk, it brings me back to all the late nights studying, hours of volunteer work, med school applications and personal statements; my hands shaking as I opened the envelope to find an acceptance letter (after several rejections). I remember all the doctors I shadowed telling me *not* to become a doctor, but I didn't listen. I wanted it. And here I am.

FOCUS ON THE POSITIVES

If you can't love everything about the work you do, you can find *something* to love about what you do. Job satisfaction isn't always inherent to the actual work, but may come from what the work brings you or allows you to do. In Medscape's survey, "Making good money at a job I like," ranked as the fourth most rewarding aspect of being a physician.

Yes, we spent a ton of money going through med school and probably have a monthly loan payment equivalent to that of a luxury car, but our earning potential is greater than much of the population. Our job situation is also pretty secure. It would be very surprising if we ever have difficulty finding work.

So, making money is definitely something to love about being a physician, but not just what's in your bank account, but what we *can do* with that money! Vacation, a nice car, early retirement... pick your dream and while you are slogging away at work, visualize that happy time when you will be on the beach in Fiji, cruising home in your sports car or comfortably retired.

We can also take time for vacation and continuing medical education. It makes me sad to think that 25% of Americans go without any vacation days at all. Our job generally allows us to take time off for family vacations and travel. We also have the option of cutting back on expenses so that we can work part-time or take a three-day weekend if that is important to us.

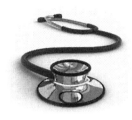

CHAPTER FIFTY-TWO
ROCK STAR PHYSICIAN PRACTICE OPTIONS

THE EMPLOYED OUT-PATIENT PHYSICIAN

Most physicians practice solo or in private, community-based groups, with more than half having an ownership interest in their practice. However, the tide is turning towards employed practice, with 26% of physicians employed by hospitals in 2013, and the trend seems to indicate an increase in employed physicians. [128]

WHY ARE HOSPITALS EMPLOYING PHYSICIANS?

The primary hospital motivation for employing physicians is to gain market share. Physician employment increases hospital admissions, diagnostic testing, and outpatient services, as well as increasing primary care referrals to employed specialists.[129]

Interestingly, hospitals lose money when they first employ physicians - $150,000 to $250,000 per year over the first 3 years as a new physician establishes a practice or adapts to new management. After the initial three years, hospitals begin to make money when they account for the value of all care, tests, and referrals generated. In fact, primary care physicians generate more annual revenue for hospitals than specialists do. [130]

Another reason that hospitals are hiring physicians is in response to health care reform. Hospital executives feel that integrating the hospital with the physician through physician employment may help them deal with Medicare payment reforms such as bundled payments, accountable care organizations (ACOs), and penalties for hospital readmissions.[131]

WHY ARE PHYSICIANS CHOOSING TO BE EMPLOYED BY HOSPITALS?

In a Jackson Health Care survey of employed physicians, the majority of respondents indicated that they chose employment because they didn't want to deal with the hassle or the business aspects of running a medical practice. Also, younger doctors tend to value better work–life balance and are more willing than preceding generations to trade income for the lifestyle flexibility provided by hospital employment.

There is a trade-off to sacrificing the autonomy of private practice for an employment model. Because of different perspectives, physicians and executives tend to see each other in an adversarial position, increasing frustration levels.[132]

One of the challenges of working for a hospital system is that government payments to hospitals are now being tied to patient satisfaction, including satisfaction with physician care. This has resulted in the use of surveys like the HCAHPS (Hospital Consumer Assessment of Healthcare Providers and Systems) survey to measure patients' perceptions of their hospital experience.[133] These surveys are a source of a great deal of stress for physicians, who often feel that they are being judged unfairly and forced to acquiesce to unreasonable expectations in order to "pass" the survey.

Interestingly, a government-sponsored study of HCAHPS was quite reserved and noncommittal in its endorsement of the project, as physician ratings did not correlate with improved outcomes.[134]

Yet this is how we are being judged. Sigh.

HCAHPS FOR PHYSICIANS

Despite limited data as above, physicians are being rated on HCAHPS survey results. Physicians that work as hospital employees need to learn how to negotiate these surveys. Paul Marsolek, an expert on hospital patient satisfaction, counsels doctors: "Forget the questions - focus on the answers." He reminds us that HCAHPS has three questions that pertain directly to physicians:

1. During this hospital stay how often did doctors treat you with courtesy and respect?

2. During this hospital stay how often did doctors listen carefully to you?

3. During this hospital stay how often did doctors explain things in a way you could understand?

The bottom line to receive an "always" response to these three questions is to be courteous and respectful, listen and demonstrate listening, and explain well to create understanding. HCAHPS doesn't care about anything else. Fortunately, these are all attributes that the Rock Star physician has in spades!

THE EMPLOYMENT CONTRACT

Since many physicians are choosing employment, we need to learn to be business-savvy, especially as it pertains to our compensation. "Negotiate your salary; this is a big mistake that new doctors make, especially women," advises Dr. Nabors, who has successfully negotiated salaries with hospital organizations. "Always aim high – know your value by finding out what other people are paying – talk to other doctors at conferences, check on-line or in the MGMA publications--and always leave room for negotiation."

Dr. Jennifer Keehbauch agrees. "I wish I had gotten more written down in my contract, rather than by verbal agreement. A lot of things that were verbal didn't materialize."

Negotiating is tough for new docs. Think about it: "You beg to get into medical school and residency, and then suddenly you change gears and have power. It's a way different mode to be in," says Dr. Ariel Cole. "Eventually you learn what you want and go after it."

I polled a group of 21 multi-specialty physicians, and slightly more than half of the doctors reported that they did not negotiate their first job salary. Interestingly, women and men reported equal likeliness of negotiating.

ROCK STAR TIP:

Negotiating experts suggest always asking for more money – respectfully, of course. The physician can negotiate not only for salary, but also for vacation, signing bonuses, and CME money.

PARTICIPATING IN HOSPITAL/EMPLOYER ACTIVITIES

When you are a Rock Star physician, you are in major demand. Not just from your patients, but from your employer or corporate entity. You will be asked to serve on various committees, take on an EHR champion role, serve as the medical director for the hospital's pet projects, teach rotating students, drop everything to see the CEO's sick kid, attend meetings, you name it. And surprise, surprise - you won't usually be compensated for these activities.

Naturally, the more you say 'yes' to these extra responsibilities (because like most doctors, you are a 'people-pleaser'), the more you are asked to participate. It becomes a vicious cycle. Eventually you may become bitter and burned out.

On the other hand, if you don't agree to participate in your employer's requests, you may be seen as not a team player. Eventually you get a bad reputation or lose support from the higher-ups.

So, how much should you contribute to your employer, outside of basic job responsibilities? Clearly a little give-and-take makes sense - if you know your limits.

Carlos Portu, MD, Internal Medicine specialist, serves both as Vice-Chairman of Medicine at his local hospital and as a board member for the outpatient medical group. "I feel more connected," he says, "and I kind of enjoy the administrative aspects. I think if I just stuck to my office work my job satisfaction would be less."

While he does receive some compensation for his roles, "the amount of work doesn't equal the compensation. But I feel that it pays off in knowing what is going to happen, getting clued into future long term strategic plans, and sometimes being in the right place at the right time can really benefit you as a physician."

Dr. Portu points out that as physicians, we tend to have an urge to participate - "we're builders, we like to build things. We often have an entrepreneurial instinct, but as an employee it's not possible unless you serve in an administrative function."

On the other hand Dr. Portu does admit that he feels burned out sometimes. "At times I feel it's almost unfair the way we're expected to do things for [the corporation] for nothing." However, the additional leverage and information makes up for the negatives for Dr. Portu.

To strike the right balance with administration, Dr. Doug Meuser suggests, "Always be professional, and don't take it personally if you aren't always understood. I try to remember that my job is to take great care of my patients, and if I can improve the level of understanding of what I do to the administration, that's a bonus."

PHYSICIAN JOBS - BECOMING A HOSPITALIST

Hospital medicine is the fastest growing medical specialty in the United States, with many Internal and Family Medicine residencies adding hospitalist tracks to their programs. The median salary for a hospitalist was $220,000 in 2012, higher than the average outpatient primary care physician ($177-194,000 for Family and Internal Medicine doctors).

"Quite a few of our graduating residents go on to become Hospitalists," says Dr. Ariel Cole, Faculty Member and Geriatric Fellowship Director for the Florida Hospital Family Medicine Residency Program. "For some of them it's a comfortable transition from residency. For others I think that the attraction comes from only being responsible for their shift, and then they are done – they don't have to totally live their job, and it gives more life-work balance."

BEING YOUR OWN BOSS

Dr. Ed Douglas, a solo Family Physician, is happy to be his own boss: "One of the reasons I wanted to be a doctor was to have my own practice. An established system is difficult to change; a large established system is almost impossible to change! So I wanted to start off the right way to begin with."

While he acknowledges that the biggest negative is money, "I still make a good and satisfying income, even though it's less than if I were employed working in the typical assembly line office. I was happy to trade a nice paycheck so I could have freedom to do things my way. A private practice isn't for everyone, particularly in today's healthcare environment. But for me at least being free and my own boss is important. Doing work I enjoy makes it fun, not work."

Having just transitioned into more of a solo-type practice, I will admit that I am happier practicing medicine than I ever have been before. Although my situation is a bit unique in that I work under the umbrella of an Urgent Care, I have the flexibility and freedom that I never had in a completely employed group setting. And while like Dr. Douglas I also took a bit of a pay cut, regaining the joy in medicine more than compensates.

SMALL GROUP PRACTICE

While there may be power in numbers, particularly in regards to insurance contracts, there are many positives to smaller group practice. The key is to find partners that share similar practice philosophies and styles. You have to be able to count on your colleagues to cover for you while you are out of the office, and share management responsibilities if you are a partner in the group.

I recently joined a small group by partnering with an Urgent Care. I provide primary care services, but when I am not in the office, the Urgent Care physicians provide coverage for acute visits for my patients. Since the Urgent Care is open seven days per week, I feel confident that my patients will be cared for, and I am able to follow-up on any urgent care visits when I'm back in the office. This structure allows me the opportunity to create my own weekly schedule and take more time away from the office without feeling that I am abandoning my patients. In turn, it increases volume to the urgent care – a mutually beneficial and highly satisfying arrangement.

ACADEMIC MEDICINE

Dr. Ariel Cole joined the faculty of her Family Medicine residency program as the Geriatric Fellowship Director. "I love geriatrics – I love their stories; hearing the living history. I also really enjoy the challenge. Although it can be frustrating, geriatric care is not cookbook – you get to use your brain."

Jennifer Keehbauch, MD, has been on faculty at her program for the last 12 years. She loves how the experience has allowed her to grow and change as a professional. "I have recreated myself many times – probably every 3-5 years," says Dr. Jennifer Keehbauch. "First I was a young faculty member, then the director of research. I developed an underserved program, became a CME director, and now I'm a hospitalist. I keep changing who I am."

"DIRECT PATIENT CARE (DPC)" OR THE MICROPRACTICE

Direct Primary Care is a relatively new practice model which charges patients a retainer fee, usually somewhere between $50-150 per month, to provide the patient comprehensive medical care.[135] This model has been gaining popularity, especially as a cost saving measure for patients with very high deductible plans. Doctors who promote the DPC model tout lower overhead costs (no insurance billing), which allows the physician to spend more time with a smaller number of patients and still be compensated fairly.

There are many other possible employment opportunities for physicians. Other practice models include concierge or "boutique" medicine, occupational medicine, urgent care work or even locum tenens. Why not travel the country--or even the world as part of your job?

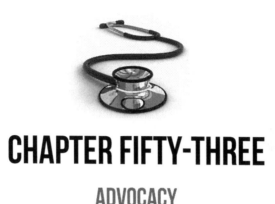

CHAPTER FIFTY-THREE

ADVOCACY

Now that you have the tools to be a Rock Star physician, you are perfectly placed to advocate for your specialty and your patients. This can be as simple as sending an email to your congressperson about a health-related bill or attending your local medical society meeting. Or even better, you can join your state or national medical societies to participate more actively in the political process.

I had the opportunity to attend the Family Medicine Congressional Conference (FMCC) in DC a few years ago, and it was an incredibly eye-opening experience. I was stunned to learn how little our elected representatives really know about what we do as physicians.

During visits to our elected officials, I watched lobbyists go in and out, each representing their own special interests. When it was our turn, we advocated for our role as physicians – and were shocked at the many questions and misunderstandings that congressional staff had about what exactly we do on a daily basis for our patients.

The challenge is that we are so busy caring for our patients that we don't have time to participate in these political maneuverings that are essential in today's health care climate. But if we don't advocate for ourselves directly, there are many other political forces ready to push their own agendas. Or, as Ajoy Kumar, MD, a faculty member at Bayfront Family Health Center and Florida Academy of Family Physicians delegate reminds us: "If you are not at the table, you are most certainly on the menu."

One of the ways that we can also advocate is through the use of Political Action Committees (PAC). Rather than taking the time out of our schedule to travel to the state capitol or DC ourselves, the PAC sponsors lobbyists to carry our message to elected representatives, and donates towards the campaigns of those who take an interest in promoting our health care agenda.

I will admit that I never felt a strong pull towards participating in the American Medical Association (AMA) or any other PAC. The groups never seemed to represent my interests or add any value to my day-to-day life. It wasn't until an early mentor of mine, Dr. Ajoy Kumar pointed out: "How can you change the policies unless you're part of the group?" that I considered taking a more active role.

"Change does not occur screaming from the outside," Dr. Kumar explained. "It takes your passion, persistence, and hard work from the inside. Get engaged in a positive manner, as failure to get engaged has its consequences too."

The reality of politics is that donating money gets your foot in the door and gets your story told. And there is power in numbers. According to the FMCC, if every Family Physician donated just $100 per year, the group would have the most powerful medical PAC in the United States.

Of course as a donating member to a PAC, you will want to listen in or participate in discussions regarding the message that your group sends to the government or even consider becoming a policy-writer yourself. It's all possible, but it starts with a single step.

Dr. Kumar elaborates: "It is not enough that you, as a family physician, advocate for your patient in this day and age in American medicine, but you must also advocate for yourself and your specialty so that you can continue to provide the quality care your patients need and deserve."

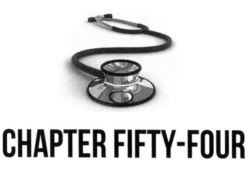

CHAPTER FIFTY-FOUR

CONCLUSION

Physician burnout is a serious problem, and is only expected to rise as doctors feel more and more beat-down by the current health care system. But burnout is not inevitable! Following the Rock Star rules will empower you as a physician, allowing you to regain the enthusiasm that you started with in medical school. Physicians need to be empowered, so that we can provide the outstanding care that our patients deserve and can then find happiness within the practice of medicine and in our personal lives.

THE ROCK STAR RULES:

1. ANYTIME YOU ARE WITH A PATIENT, REMEMBER THAT YOU ARE ON-STAGE.

The most important rule of the Rock Star physician is to play the part and play it well. When you are on-stage, you must portray the image of an ideal doctor – affable, confident, and caring, even when you're not feeling your best. Practice acting the part, constantly remembering that any time you are in front of a patient (or staff member, or colleague), you are on-stage. Not only does this benefit your patients, but it benefits yourself as well. As you practice acting like a Rock Star, you will actually become one. And while remembering to stay on-stage is the key to clinical success, getting off-stage efficiently is the solution to preventing burnout and finding happiness as a physician.

2. WHEN IN DOUBT, ASK YOURSELF: "IS THIS IN THE BEST INTEREST OF MY PATIENT(S)?"

The bottom line in becoming a successful physician, and especially a Rock Star physician, is *never to lose patient focus.* You will never go wrong if you ask yourself: "Is this decision in the best interest of my patient(s)?" However, in order to best care for our patients, we also have to consider what is in *our own* best interest as physicians. An empowered and enthusiastic physician is much more able to provide top quality care than someone who is burned out and miserable.

Sometimes we have to make choices as physicians that may *seem* to be detrimental to our patients, like cutting back on office hours, or not taking telephone calls in the middle of the night. But in fact, prioritizing our own quality of life will actually allow us to serve *more* patients, with more caring and probably for a longer career period of time.

3. BE AVAILABLE.

The Rock Star must have an audience, and office availability is the core of patient satisfaction and financial success. Being available means having plenty of office slots to work-in your concerned or ill patients, on the same day if at all possible. Schedule frequent follow-up visits for your patients and don't hesitate to bring them into the office for any medical needs, paperwork, forms, etc. Since the Rock Star physician uses techniques to minimize time spent on non-direct patient care, he is always available to see his patients during office hours.

However, even the Rock Star physician cannot (and should not) be available every second of the day. We must take time for our own mental well-being and that includes time away from the office. The Rock Star doctor arranges with a trusted colleague or urgent care center to provide coverage when necessary, always following up with her patients when she returns to the office.

4. LISTEN TO YOUR PATIENTS

Listening is so simple and is ultimately the backbone of clinical success. A few extra minutes (or even six seconds!) will transform you into a Rock Star physician that patients love to see, while giving you the information that you need to make correct clinical assessments. Spending time listening actually shortens the total amount of time that we spend in the office, while making it seem to the patient that the visit was much longer. Remember that we heal as much by listening and caring as much as by the strength of our prescription pads.

5. LEARN HOW TO SHOW EMPATHY

Even on your worst day, you can still to put on a smile or an expression of concern and demonstrate empathy. Putting yourself in your patient's shoes makes all the difference, even if you have to "fake it 'til you make it!" Showing empathy is especially important to succeed with your most challenging patients.

Just *acting* empathetic has been shown to translate into true feelings of empathy and is something that can be learned and practiced. The more you practice showing empathy, the easier it becomes to truly feel empathy, which in turn leads to less stress and burnout in the physician.

6. MAKE THE 'PROBLEM LIST' YOUR BEST FRIEND

Instead of torturing yourself clicking or paging through a thick medical chart, creating a refined problem list will allow you to use clinical time efficiently and effectively. Spending the extra time needed to create a really great problem list will improve your productivity immensely during office visits and allow you to focus on the patient's needs rather than the chart.

7. LEARN TO DOCUMENT AN EXAM JUST BY LOOKING

The Rock Star physician saves time where she can. An extremely directed physical examination is often medically appropriate and should be instituted whenever possible. A simple touch on the hand, elbow, or shoulder, or checking your patients pulse while you talk with them may be all that you need to do to make a physical connection, without spending unnecessary time on non-useful or invasive exams.

8. HEALTH MAINTENANCE: EVERY VISIT, EVERY TIME.

Taking the opportunity to update health maintenance at every office visit is a true Rock Star move. All patients deserve to receive essential evidence-based preventive care, even when they don't schedule a "routine" wellness visit. The Rock Star physician, using an excellent problem list, will take a moment to review essential preventive care services like cancer screening even during visits for chronic disease management or acute illness care.

9. MAXIMIZE PATIENT-PHYSICIAN FACE-TO-FACE TIME

The Rock Star physician must prevent anything that reduces face-to-face time with his patients. This focus on the physician-patient relationship is really the core of the medical profession, increasing patient and physician satisfaction. Avoiding non-clinical responsibilities by delegating to others or by creating templates and forms will maximize your profitability and decrease burnout.

10. YOU DON'T NEED TO KNOW ALL THE ANSWERS, JUST WHERE TO FIND THEM

Despite our minimum of 11 years and 20,000 plus hours of training, we just don't know it all. Heck, we don't even know the tip of the iceberg. Maybe that's what makes us good —we acknowledge that we *don't* know it all and continually strive to improve our knowledge and thus the care of our patients. Creating customizable tools and resources that are available at your fingertips optimizes the office visit experience. Having your computer loaded with the latest EBM-guidelines will wow your patients with your clinical acumen, while speeding your office visit.

11. DON'T SELL YOURSELF SHORT!

Throughout our years of training, we became accustomed to sacrificing our own happiness to care for our patients. We suffered from lack of sleep, deferred time with friends and family, and delayed our income potential as we slogged through those low-paying residency years. And, all the while watched our student loans tick ever upwards with compounding interest.

It's time to stand up for ourselves! As Rock Star physicians, we serve as advocates for our patients; we educate our communities, and we train the future of medicine. We must advocate not only for our patients, but also for ourselves as physicians.

We need to ensure that we are adequately compensated for our professional services by coding correctly and avoiding nonclinical tasks. We also need to focus on the bigger picture of politics and government in health care by speaking up for our profession and making our message heard to our elected representatives.

12. MAKE YOUR MENTAL HEALTH A PRIORITY

Although this is the last rule, it may be the most important. Maintaining your own mental and physical health to find work-life balance is absolutely essential, and the core of the Rock Star physician. As role models not only to our patients, but also to the future generation of physicians, it is our responsibility to remove the stigma of seeking psychological care and to emphasize the importance of continual self-growth and nurturing. We must turn our mission of helping and healing inwards and prioritize our own mental health and work-life balance for the good of ourselves and our patients.

Remember, you're not only a physician. You are a Rock Star physician.

ACKNOWLEDGEMENTS

I would never in a million years have finished this book without the guidance and support of my Rock Star editor (a patient *and* a friend) Newt Barrett. His constant encouragement (including emails like "Are you my noncompliant author?") gave me the motivation to finish a project that has been three years in the making. He walked me through every step of the process, and provided invaluable guidance and support.

This book would not have been possible without the input from many Rock Star physicians, as listed in the biography of contributors. Dr. Douglas Meuser, my residency advisor, first inspired the idea of being on-stage and supplied hours of helpful information.

Dr. Jennifer Keehbauch, a mentor and inspiration since my 4th year medical school externship, provided valuable insight and assistance during the editing process.

My dear friends Roberta Chung, MD, and Emily Nabors, MD, with whom I bonded during our painful residency years, shared their insights as Rock Star physicians and provided the difficult and honest feedback that I truly needed.My current employer Rob McGann, a journalist in his previous life, painstakingly reviewed the manuscript for formatting issues and provided recommendations on writing technique.

I thank the many practicing physicians who read the manuscript and provided me with feedback: Jay Lee, MD, Elizabeth Shandor, DO,

Charles Neal, MD, Easton Jackson, MD, and Ed Douglas, DO. Megan Janson, MD, provided me with feedback from a resident perspective, as did Anisha Patel, a 4th year medical student. Steve Cohen, PsyD, added valuable insight as a psychologist who cares for many physicians. I thank Ashley Law for reading the manuscript and for being an amazing office manager.

Much of this book was inspired by Paul Marsolek, a patient satisfaction hospital administrator who worked with me at Physicians Regional. He often pointed out (at large group meetings, to my embarrassment) how my practice succeeded in providing top patient satisfaction, and told me that he used me as an example when lecturing to physician groups.

And of course, I thank my wonderful patients, who have allowed me into their lives. I especially want to acknowledge Bob Lang, who inspired the title of this book by calling me a Rock Star in his patient satisfaction survey.

BIOGRAPHY OF CONTRIBUTORS

Roberta Chung, MD. Family Physician. Orlando, FL.

Ariel Cole, MD, FAAFP, CAQ Geriatrics. Director Geriatric Fellowship Florida Hospital, Orlando, FL.

Ed Douglas, DO, Family Physician. Private practice Springfield, MO.

Alan Falkoff, MD. Family Physician, Stamford, CT. Connecticut's Best Family Physicians award.

Carrie Gittings, MD, Family Physician. Lee Memorial Health Systems Community Health; FSU adjunct faculty member.

John Gross, MD, Family Physician, St. Petersburg, FL. Medical director of St. Anthony's Primary Care.

Easton Jackson, MD, Family Physician. Private practice, West Valley City, UT

Jennifer Keehbauch, MD. Family Physician, Orlando, FL. Florida Hospital Family Medicine Residency Program faculty, 2007 Family Physician of the Year, 2014 President of the Florida Academy of Family Physicians.

Ajoy Kumar, MD, Family Physician. St. Petersburg, FL. Residency Faculty, AMA delegate

Paul Marsolek, Director of Loyalty and Engagement, Director of Performance Improvement at Health Management Associates, Published Author of books on health care leadership.

Douglas Meuser, MD. Family Physician. FSU College of Medicine faculty member, UCF Student Health physician, medical director of the Athletic Training Educational Program at UCF, and Family Medicine Faculty of the Year winner.

Emily Nabors, MD. Family Physician. Private practice, Morrisville, NC. 2010 Most Influential Woman. 2011 Patient's Choice Award.

Charles Neal, MD, Family Physician. Mt. Vernon, IL.

Beth Shandor, DO, Internal Medicine, Philadelphia, PA.

Carlos Portu, MD, Internal Medicine. Marco Island, FL. Published Naples Daily News newspaper series "White Coat Notes," 2012 Physicians Regional Healthcare System Physician of the Year.

David Voran, MD. Family Physician, private practice Platte City, MO.

ENDNOTES

1   http://www.medscape.com/viewarticle/838437_7

2   *Arch Intern Med.* 2012; 172(18):1377-1385. doi:10.1001/ archinternmed.2012.3199.

3   A RAND Corporation study (Retail Clinic Visits and Receipt of Primary Care
Published in: Journal of General Internal Medicine, v. 28, no. 4, Apr. 2013, p. 504-512

4   Annals of Family MedicineTime Spent in Face-to-Face Patient Care and Work Outside the Examination Room Andrew Gottschalk, BS, Susan A. Flocke, PhD Ann Fam Med. 2005;3(6):488-493.

5   http://www.ncbi.nlm.nih.gov/pmc/articles/PMC539473/ J R Soc Med. May 2003; 96(5): 219–222.

6   http://www.ama-assn.org/resources/doc/ama-foundation/ healthlitclinicians.pdf

7   **Mayo Clinic Proceedings** Volume 81, Issue 3 , Pages 338-344, March 2006 Patients' Perspectives on Ideal Physician Behaviors Neeli M. Bendapudi, PhD, et al http://www.mayoclinicproceedings.org/article/S0025-6196(11)61463-8/ abstract

8   Communication Practices of Physicians with High Patient
    Satisfaction Ratings, Tallman, et al. Perm J. 2007 Winter; 11
    (1): 19-29 www.ncbi.nlm.nih.gov/pmc/articles/PMC3061374/

9   How Do Distress and Well-being Relate to Medical Student
    Empathy? A Multicenter Study http://link.springer.com/
    article/10.1007/s11606-006-0039-6

10 September 2009 - Volume 84 - Issue 9 - pp 1182-1191 doi:
    10.1097/ACM.0b013e3181b17e55 The Devil is in the Third
    Year: A Longitudinal Study of Erosion of Empathy in Medical
    School Hojat, Mohammadreza PhD; Vergare, Michael J. MD;
    Maxwell, Kaye; Brainard, George PhD; Herrine, Steven K.
    MD; Isenberg, Gerald A. MD; Veloski, Jon MS; Gonnella,
    Joseph S. MD http://journals.lww.com/academicmedicine/
    Abstract/2009/09000/The_Devil_is_in_the_Third_Year__A_
    Longitudinal.12.aspx

11 Front Hum Neurosci. 2013; 7: 233. 2013 Jun 11. doi: 10.3389/
    fnhum.2013.00233

12 Differences in medical students' empathy. Newton, Bruce W.;
    Savidge, Mildred A.; Barber, Laurie; Cleveland, Elton; Clardy,
    James; Beeman, Gail; Hart, Thomas Academic Medicine, Vol
    75(12), Dec 2000, 1215

13 Mayo Clinic Proceedings Volume 80, Issue 12, December 2005,
    Pages 1613–1622
    Liselotte N. Dyrbye, MD http://www.sciencedirect.com/science/
    article/pii/S0025619611610574

14 (Students lose empathy for patients during medical school
    By MYRLE CROASDALE — Posted March 24, 2008
    Amednews.com

15 Striking a balance: Training medical students to provide
    empathetic care. Rosenfield, Paul J.; Jones, Lee Medical
    Education, Vol 38(9), Sep 2004, 927-933. doi: 10.1111/j.1365-

2929.2004.01931.x http://psycnet.apa.org/index.cfm?fa=search. displayRecord&uid=2004-17982-002

16 Montague E, Chen P, Xu J, Chewning B, Barrett B. Nonverbal interpersonal interactions in clinical encounters and patient perceptions of empathy. J Participat Med. 2013 Aug 14; 5:e33. http://www.jopm.org/evidence/research/2013/08/14/nonverbal-interpersonal-interactions-in-clinical-encounters-and-patient-perceptions-of-empathy/

17 http://www.ncbi.nlm.nih.gov/pmc/articles/PMC1494899/ What is Clinical Empathy? J Gen Intern Med. Aug 2003; 18(8): 670–674.

18 Differences in medical students' empathy. http://psycnet.apa.org/psycinfo/2000-14369-001 Newton, Bruce W.; Savidge, Mildred A.; Barber, Laurie; Cleveland, Elton; Clardy, James; Beeman, Gail; Hart, Thomas Academic Medicine, Vol 75(12), Dec 2000, 1215. doi: 10.1097/00001888-200012000-00020

19 Dr. Fleeson, Wake Forest University, Journal of Personality 2012

20 http://www.aafp.org/dam/AAFP/documents/news/NP-Kit-FP-NP-UPDATED.pdf

21 Asia Pacific Family MedicineJanuary 2014, 13:2,Importance of physicians' attire: factors influencing the impression it makes on patients, a cross-sectional study Hiroshi Kurihara, et al

22 The Permanente Journal Kaiser Permanente Communication Practices of Physicians With High Patient-Satisfaction Ratings Karen Tallman, PhD, Tom Janisse, MD, [...], and John T Hsu, MD, MBA, MSCE

23 http://www.gallup.com/poll/1654/honesty-ethics-professions.aspx#4

24 ETHICS IN MEDICINE University of Washington School of Medicine
https://depts.washington.edu/bioethx/topics/truth.html

25 Primary Care Companion to The Journal of Clinical Psychiatry. Lies in the Doctor-Patient Relationship John J. Palmieri, MD and Theodore A. Stern, MD http://www.ncbi.nlm.nih.gov/pmc/articles/PMC2736034/

26 Apology in Medical Practice: An Emerging Clinical Skill Aaron Lazare, MD, *JAMA.* 2006;296(11):1401-1404. doi:10.1001/jama.296.11.1401.

27 Journal of General Internal Medicine - Physician Respect for Patients with Obesity Mary Margaret Huizinga, MD, MPH, Lisa A. Cooper, MD, MPH, [...], and Mary Catherine Beach, MD, MPH http://www.ncbi.nlm.nih.gov/pmc/articles/PMC2771236/ Thoroughness

28 Are physicians' attitudes of respect accurately perceived by patients and associated with more positive communication behaviors? Mary Catherine Beacha, Debra L. Roterd, Nae-Yuh Wanga,, Patrick S. Dugganb, Lisa A. Coopera, http://www.sciencedirect.com/science/article/pii/S0738399106001868

29 Environ Health Perspect. Oct 2011; 119(10): a426–a427.

30 Identifying the Causes of Staff TurnoverJudy Capko *Fam Pract Manag.* **2001 Apr;8(4)**:29-33

31 Does the "Office Nurse" Level of Training Matter in the Family Medicine Office Erickson, et al doi:10.3122/jabfm.2012.06.110138J Am Board Fam MedNovember-December 2012 vol. 25 no. 6 854-861
Demonstrating the Value of the RN in Ambulatory Care Beth Ann Swan, et al Econ. 2006;24(6):315-322

32 Demonstrating the Value of the RN in Ambulatory Care Beth Ann Swan, et al Econ. 2006;24(6):315-322

33   Envisioning New Roles for Medical Assistants: Strategies From Patient-Centered Medical Homes Dana Naughton, et al *Fam Pract Manag.* 2013 Mar-Apr;20(2):7-12.

34   Understanding Medical Assistant Practice Liability Issues Carolyn Buppert Dermatology Nursing. 2008;20(4):327-329

35   LPN Scope of Practice White Paper 2005, https://www.ncsbn.org/Final_11_05_Practical_Nurse_Scope_Practice_White_Paper.pdf

36   Keys to High-Functioning Office Teams Anton J. Kuzel, MD, MHPE *Fam Pract Manag.* 2011 May- June;18(3):1518.

37   How Many Staff Members Do You Need?Crystal S. Reeves, CPC *Fam Pract Manag.* 2002 Sep;9(8):45-49.

38   http://www.ncbi.nlm.nih.gov/pmc/articles/PMC3776508/

39   http://www.bmj.com/content/331/7531/1524

40   Fam Med 2011; 43(9) 643-7 http://www.stfm.org/fmhub/fm2011/October/William643.pdf

41   http://www.ajicjournal.org/article/S0196-6553(11)01011-X/abstract.

42   http://www.bmj.com/content/328/7438/501

43   https://articles.mercola.com/sites/articles/archive/2008/01/02/doctors-interrupt.aspx - JAMA Jan 20, 1999; 281: 283-287).

44   http://www.bmj.com/content/328/7438/501 Length of patient's monologue, rate of completion, and relation to other components of the clinical encounter: observational intervention study in primary care
      BMJ 2004; 328 doi: http://dx.doi.org/10.1136/bmj.328.7438.501 (Published 26 February 2004)

45   http://www.ncbi.nlm.nih.gov/pmc/articles/PMC3061374/

46   http://www.ncbi.nlm.nih.gov/pmc/articles/PMC3061374/

47 http://www.uspreventiveservicestaskforce.org

48 http://www.aafp.org/fpm/2009/0900/p12.html

49 Communication Practices of Physicians With High Patient-Satisfaction Ratings Karen Tallman, PhD, Tom Janisse, MD, [...], and John T Hsu, MD, MBA, MSCE http://www.ncbi.nlm.nih.gov/pmc/articles/PMC3061374/

50 CMAJ. May 1, 1995; 152(9): 1423–1433.Effective physician-patient communication and health outcomes: a review.M A Stewart http://www.ncbi.nlm.nih.gov/pmc/articles/PMC1337906/?page=11

51 "The Enduring Impact of What Clinicians Say to People with Low Back Pain;" Darlow et al, Ann Fam Med 2013; 11 (6): 527-534

52 http://www.cms.gov/Outreach-and-Education/Medicare-Learning-Network-MLN/MLNProducts/downloads/AWV_Chart_ICN905706.pdf

53 http://medicaleconomics.modernmedicine.com/medical-economics/news/how-manufacturing-process-transformed-healthcare-delivery

54 http://profitable-practice.softwareadvice.com/value-stream-mapping-to-improve-workflow-0114/

55 http://qualitysafety.bmj.com/content/21/1/47.long

56 http://www.acponline.org/running_practice/practice_management/education/practice_efficiency.pdf

57 https://www.scopeofpain.com/tools-resources/

58 http://www.justice.gov/dea/druginfo/ds.shtml

59   Frequency of Failure to Inform Patients of Clinically Significant Outpatient Test Results Lawrence P. Casalino, MD et al *Arch Intern Med.* 2009;169(12):1123-1129. doi:10.1001/archinternmed.2009.130. http://archinte.jamanetwork.com/article.aspx?articleid=415120

60   Management of Laboratory Test Results in Family Practice *J Fam Pract.* 2000 August;49(08):1-8. James W. Mold, MD et al http://www.jfponline.com/home/article/management-of-laboratory-test-results-in-family-practice/6bf8fa1cb56cafb1cd7fde711feef78b.html

61   The Impact of Prior Authorization Requirements on Primary Care Physicians' Offices: Report of Two Parallel Network Studies J Am Board Fam Med May 1, 2013 26:340

62   http://medicaleconomics.modernmedicine.com/medical-economics/news/curing-prior-authorization-headache?page=full

63   http://www.americangeriatrics.org/files/documents/beers/2012BeersCriteria_JAGS.pdf

64   Ann Fam Med. Nov 2005; 3(6): 488–493. Andrew Gottschalk, BS[1] and Susan A. Flocke, PhD[2] http://www.ncbi.nlm.nih.gov/pmc/articles/PMC1466945/#__ffn_sectitle

65   http://www.aafp.org/fpm/2004/0700/p43.html Should You Charge Your Patients for "Free" Services? Leigh Ann Backer *Fam Pract Manag.* 2004 Jul-Aug;11(7):43-53

66   http://www.ncbi.nlm.nih.gov/pmc/articles/PMC3061374/

67   The Associated Press/Ipsos Poll: Almost A Third Of Americans Say Paying For Drugs Is A Problem In Their Families

68   Cost-Related Medication Underuse Among Chronically Ill Adults: the Treatments People Forgo, How Often, and Who Is at Risk John D. Piette, PhD, Michele Heisler, MD, and Todd H. Wagner, PhD http://www.ncbi.nlm.nih.gov/pmc/articles/

PMC1448534/

69   Cost-Related Medication Underuse: Do Patients With Chronic
     Illnesses Tell Their Doctors? John D. Piette; Michele Heisler;
     Todd H. WagnerArch Intern Med. 2004;164(16):1749-1755.
     doi:10.1001/archinte.164.16.1749.

70   Journal of General Internal Medicine January 1996, Volume
     11, Issue 1, pp 1-8 The difficult patient Dr. Steven R. Hahn
     MD, et al http://link.springer.com/article/10.1007/BF02603477

71   http://www.biomedcentral.com/1472-6963/6/128 BMC Health
     Services Research 2006

72   The Patient-Physician Relationship and Medical Utilization Denis
     J. Lynch, Ph.D., et al http://www.ncbi.nlm.nih.gov/pmc/articles/
     PMC2018838/

73   Mental Illness Statistics - The Kim Foundation http://www.
     thekimfoundation.org/html/about_mental_ill/statistics.html

74   Western Journal of Medicine, BMJ Group The poor physical
     health of people with mental illness David P J Osborn, http://
     www.ncbi.nlm.nih.gov/pmc/articles/PMC1071612/

75   Somatoform Disorders OLIVER OYAMA, PhD, et al, Florida
     Am Fam Physician. 2007 Nov 1;76(9):1333-1338 http://www.
     aafp.org/afp/2007/1101/p1333.html

76   Physicians Postgraduate Press, Inc. On Clinicians' Professional
     Difficulties Frank V. deGruy, M.D., M.S.F.M.

77   Somatization: Diagnosing it sooner through emotion-focused
     interviewing J Fam Pract. 2005 March;54(03):231-243. http://
     www.jfponline.com/fileadmin/jfp_archive/pdf/5403/5403JFP_
     AppliedEvidence2.pdf
     Allan Abbass, MD, FRCPC Faculty of Medicine, Dalhousie
     University Halifax,Nova Scotia

78   Psychosom Med. 2002 Mar-Apr;64(2):258-66.The PHQ-15:

validity of a new measure for evaluating the severity of somatic symptoms. Kroenke K[1], Spitzer RL, Williams JB.

79   J Psychosom Res. 2010 Jun;68(6):521-33. doi: 10.1016/j. jpsychores.2009.10.012. Epub 2010 Jan 15. Effect of psychiatric consultation models in primary care. A systematic review and meta-analysis of randomized clinical trials.van der Feltz-Cornelis CM[1], Van Os TW, Van Marwijk HW, Leentjens AF. http://www. ncbi.nlm.nih.gov/pubmed/20488268

80   Gen Hosp Psychiatry. 1994 Nov;16(6):381-7.Effectiveness of psychiatric intervention with somatization disorder patients: improved outcomes at reduced costs.Rost K[1], Kashner TM, Smith RG Jr. http://www.ncbi.nlm.nih.gov/pubmed/7843574

81   Efficacy of treatment for somatoform disorders: a review of randomized controlled trials. Kroenke K. http://www.ncbi.nlm. nih.gov/pubmed/18040099

82   Population based study of fatigue and psychological distress BMJ 1994; 308 doi: http://dx.doi.org/10.1136/ bmj.308.6931.763 (Published 19 March 1994)

83   Prevalence of Fatigue and Chronic Fatigue Syndrome in a Primary Care Practice David W. Bates, MD, et al *Arch Intern Med.* 1993;153(24):2759-2765. doi:10.1001/ archinte.1993.00410240067007 http://archinte.jamanetwork. com/article.aspx?articleid=618202

84   Chronic Fatigue in Primary CarePrevalence, Patient Characteristics, and OutcomeKurt Kroenke, MD; et al *JAMA.* 1988;260(7):929-934. doi:10.1001/jama.1988. http:// jama.jamanetwork.com/article.aspx?articleid=373491

85   Journal of General Internal Medicine August 1993, Volume 8, Issue 8, pp 436-440 Psychiatric disorders and medical care utilization among people in the general population who report fatigue Dr. Edward A. Walker MD,et al

86   Canadian Family PhysicianMay 2007 vol. 53 no. 5 892

87   Advances in Psychiatric Treatment **(2000)**6: 57-64doi: 10.1192/apt.6.1.57

88   Improving Patient Communication in No TimeEllen J. Belzer, MPA *Fam Pract Manag.* 1999 May;6(5):23-28.

89   Taking Care of the Hateful Patient, James E Groves, MD; NEJM 298 (16): 883-7, 1978 April 20

90   Outliers: The story of success (309pp.). By Malcolm Gladwell. New York: Little Brown, 2008

91   http://www.aafp.org/dam/AAFP/documents/news/NP-Kit-FP-NP-UPDATED.pdf

92   Fasting Time and Lipid Levels in a Community-Based PopulationA Cross-sectional Study *Arch Intern Med.* 2012;172(22):1707-1710. doi:10.1001/archinternmed.2012.3708. http://archinte.jamanetwork.com/article.aspx?articleid=1391022
Pediatrics. 2011 Sep;128(3):463-70. doi: 10.1542/peds.2011-0844. Epub 2011 Aug 1.Fasting might not be necessary before lipid screening: a nationally representative cross-sectional study. http://www.ncbi.nlm.nih.gov/pubmed/21807697
Is fasting necessary before lipid tests? BMJ 2012; 345 doi: http://dx.doi.org/10.1136/bmj.e7662 (Published 14 November 2012) http://www.bmj.com/content/345/bmj.e7662

93   AJN, American Journal of Nursing:February 2013 - Volume 113 - Issue 2 - p 15 http://journals.lww.com/ajnonline/Fulltext/2013/02000/NewsCAP   Fasting for lipid screening may be.6.aspx

94   Medscape Family Physician Compensation Report 2014 http://www.medscape.com

95   Am J Med. 2001 Dec 21;111(9B):15S-20S.Primary care

physician attitudes regarding communication with hospitalists. Pantilat SZ[1], Lindenauer PK, Katz PP, Wachter RM. http://www.ncbi.nlm.nih.gov/pubmed/11790363

96   Hospitalists and family physicians: Understanding opportunities and risks*J Fam Pract.* 2004 June;53(06):473-481. Ann Scheck McAlearney, ScD http://www.jfponline.com/index.php?id=22143&tx_ttnews[tt_news]=167362

97   http://fojp.com/sites/default/files/InFocus_Spring13_0.pdf

98   http://www.cms.gov/Outreach-and-Education/Medicare-Learning-Network-MLN/MLNProducts/Downloads/Transitional-Care-Management-Services-Fact-Sheet-ICN908628.pdf

99   CPT only copyright 2012 American Medical Association. All rights reserved

100   Canadian Family PhysicianJanuary 2012 vol. 58 no. 152-54

101   http://www.ajemjournal.com/article/S0735-6757(13)00405-1/abstract

102   http://www.northwestern.edu/newscenter/stories/2014/01/do-doctors-spend-too-much-time-looking-at-computer-screen.html

103   http://www.modernhealthcare.com/article/20130824/MAGAZINE/308249958#

104   How to Get All the 99214s You Deserve. Emily Hill, PA-C Fam Pract Manag. 2003 Oct;10(9):31-36. http://www.aafp.org/fpm/2003/1000/p31.html

105   Coding "Routine" Office Visits: 99213 or 99214? Before choosing 99213 for routine visits, consider whether your work qualifies for a 99214. Peter R. Jensen, MD, CPC Fam Pract Manag. 2005 Sep;12(8):52-57. http://www.aafp.org/fpm/2005/0900/p52.html

106   The Painful Truth: Physicians Are Not Invincible

Merry N. Miller, MD, K. Ramsey Mcgowen, PhD, Department of Psychiatry and Behavioral Sciences, James H. Quillen College of Medicine, East Tennessee State University, Johnson City. South Med J. 2000;93(10)

107 National Review of Medicine March 2006, Vol 3, No. 5 "Doctors and DIVORCE" Gillian Woodford

108 Harv Rev Psychiatry. 2008;16(3):181-94..Prescription opioid abuse and dependence among physicians: hypotheses and treatment. Merlo LJ[1], Gold MS.

109 J Gen Intern Med. 1992 Jul-Aug;7(4):424-31.The heart of darkness: the impact of perceived mistakes on physicians. Christensen JF[1], Levinson W, Dunn PM.

110 Jt Comm J Qual Patient Saf. 2007 Aug;33(8):467-76.The emotional impact of medical errors on practicing physicians in the United States and Canada. Waterman AD et al

111 Shanafelt TD, Bradley KA, Wipf JE, Black AL: Burnout and self-reported patient care in an internal medicine residency program. *Ann Intern Med.* 2002;136(5):358-367.

112 *J Clin Outcomes Manage* 2008 May;15(5):240-247Supporting health care workers after medical error: considerations for health care leaders *White AA, Waterman AD, McCotter P, Boyle DJ, Gallagher TH*

113 BMJ. 1999 Sep 4;319(7210):605-8.Doctors as patients: postal survey examining consultants and general practitioners adherence to guidelines. Forsythe M[1], Calnan M, Wall B.

114 Western J Med Jan 2001 : 174 A qualitative study of physicians' own wellness-promotion practices Eric L Weiner, Geoffrey R Swain, [...], and Mark Gottlieb

115 D.E. Stewart, F. Ahmad, A.M. Cheung, B. Bergman, and D.L. Dell. Journal of Women's Health & Gender-Based Medicine. March 2000, 9(2): 185-190. doi:10.1089/152460900318687.

116 Soc Sci Med. 1996 Oct;43(8):1253-61.

117 Can Fam Physician. Oct 1996; 42: 1928–1935.Time spent on professional activities and unwaged domestic work. Is it different for male and female primary care physicians who have children at home? C. A. Woodward, A. P. Williams, B. Ferrier, and M. Cohen

118 Academic Medicine:August 1999 Medicine and motherhood: shifting trends among female physicians from 1922 to 1999 Potee, R A; Gerber, A J; Ickovics, J R

119 Academic Medicine:January 2011 - Volume 86 - Issue 1 - pp 43-47 Gender Differences in Academic Productivity and Leadership Appointments of Physicians Throughout Academic Careers Reed, Darcy A. MD, MPH et al

120 Differences in income between male and female primary care physicians.Wallace AE, Weeks WB Department of Psychiatry, Dartmouth Medical School, USA. Journal of the American Medical Women's Association (1972) [2002, 57(4):180-184]

121 Are Women Overinvesting in Education? Evidence from the Medical Profession M. Keith Chen, et al Journal of Human Capital Volume 6 number 2 (Summer 2012), pp. 124-149 http://www.jstor.org/stable/10.1086/665536 Stress and Women Physicians 1990, pp 129-141Female Physician Stress Marjorie A. Bowman, Deborah I. Allen

122 Psychiatric illness in female physicians. Are high rates of depression an occupational hazard? Department of Psychiatry, Washington University School of Medicine, St Louis 63110, USA. northc@psychiatry.wustl.edu Postgraduate Medicine [1997, 101(5):233-6, 239-40, 242]

123 Medical Care:November 1991 Sex Differences in Patients' and Physicians' Communication During Primary Care Medical Visits DrPH, Debra Roter; Lipkin, Mack JR MD; Korsgaard, Audrey

124 Patient Education and Counseling Volume 48, Issue 3 , Pages 217-224, December 2002 Do patients talk differently to male and female physicians? A meta-analytic review Judith A Hall Debra L Roter

125 Are patients more likely to see physicians of the same sex? Recent national trends in primary care medicine Margaret C. Fang, MD, MPH, et al http://dx.doi.org/10.1016/j.amjmed.2004.03.043

126 Journal of General Internal Medicine Volume 15, Issue 6, pages 372–380, June 2000

127 Medscape Family Physician Compensation Report 2014, Leslie Kane, Carol Peckham, April 15, 2014

128 http://www.jacksonhealthcare.com/media/191888/2013physiciantrends-void_ebk0513.pdf

129 http://www.hschange.com/CONTENT/1230/ Rising Hospital Employment of Physicians: Better Quality, Higher Costs? Issue Brief No. 136August 2011 Ann S. O'Malley, Amelia M. Bond, Robert A. Berenson

130 http://medicaleconomics.modernmedicine.com/medical-economics/news/primary-care-physicians-generate-more-revenue-hospitals-specialists?contextCategoryId=146#sthash.wEuaPkoW.dpuf

131 Hospitals' Race to Employ Physicians — The Logic behind a Money-Losing PropositionRobert Kocher, M.D., and Nikhil R. Sahni, B.S.N Engl J Med 2011; 364:1790-1793May 12, 2011 http://www.nejm.org/doi/full/10.1056/NEJMp1101959

132 Quality, lack of errors, cost containment/ profitabilityMending the Gap between Physicians and Hospital ExecutivesDeane Waldman and Kenneth H. Cohn http://healthcarecollaboration.typepad.com/healthcare_collaboration_/files/physhospgap_waldman.pdf

133 http://www.cms.gov/Medicare/Quality-Initiatives-Patient-Assessment-Instruments/HospitalQualityInits/HospitalHCAHPS.html

134 http://www.cms.gov/Medicare/Quality-Initiatives-Patient-Assessment-Instruments/HospitalQualityInits/downloads/HCAHPSCostsBenefits200512.pdf

135 http://www.aafp.org/dam/AAFP/documents/practice_management/payment/DirectPrimaryCare.pdf

FORMS

RSB001 – problem list – Sample Problem List

RSB002 – new patient handout – Sample new patient handout

RSB003 – Patient self-assessment pg. 1 – Patient self-assessment form

RSB004 – Patient self-assessment pg. 2

RSB005 – dictation template – Wellness visit dictation template

RSB006 – wellness into – Wellness visit patient information

RSB007 – screening form – Medicare screening form

RSB008 – resources – Sample health care resources

RSB009 – Transitional care – Transitional care tracking sheet

RSB010 – Emergency protocol – Sample emergency protocol

RSB011 – Billing forms – Billing and coding snapshot

Made in the USA
Lexington, KY
30 January 2018